ALCOHOL FREE

Straight Up with a Twist

A 101-Day Journey Toward Easy Sobriety
J.W. Collier

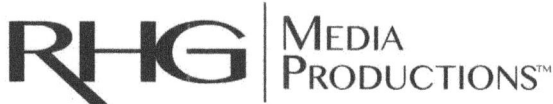

Alcohol-Free
Straight Up with a Twist:
A 101-Day Journey Toward Easy Sobriety

Copyright © 2021 by J.W. Collier

RHG Media Productions
25495 Southwick Drive #103
Hayward, CA 94544.

All rights reserved. No part of this publication may be reproduced distributed or transmitted in any form or by any means including photocopying recording or other electronic or mechanical means without proper written permission of author or publisher, except in the case of brief quotations embodied in critical reviews and certain other noncommercial uses permitted by copyright law.

ISBN 978-1-7369896-1-6 (paperback)
ISBN 978-1-7369896-0-9 (hardcover)

Visit us online at www.YourPurposeDrivenPractice.com

Printed in the United States of America.

WHAT PEOPLE ARE SAYING

"Everyone who begins a journey to stop drinking needs to feel less alone, and J.W.'s honest and vulnerable sharing and beautiful insights shine a brilliant light that illuminates the path for others."
—Annie Grace
Author of *This Naked Mind* and *The Alcohol Experiment*

"This is a powerful book that takes readers on a journey from the initial uncertainty and fear of day 1, right through to the joys of living a life without alcohol."
—Simon Chapple
Author of *The Sober Survival Guide* and *How to Quit Alcohol in 50 Days*

"I can relate to J.W. Collier's *Alcohol-Free: Straight Up with a Twist*'s story of addiction in this unique glimpse inside the mind of a functioning alcoholic willing to change his life."
—Brianne Davis
Actress, History Channel's *Six*, and author of best-selling novel *Secret Life of a Hollywood Sex & Love Addict*

"The pages are filled with wisdom and valuable, life-saving insight."
—Brittany Priestley
Author of "Mommy Drunkest"

"*Alcohol-Free* provides a unique insight not only into why someone might decide to become sober but also how to manage the inevitable emotional rollercoaster that will follow."
   —Leah Martin-Brown
   Singer-Songwriter at Evol Walks

"It's really a story of how you can change, let go of the illusion of alcohol and find real peace and authentic freedom."
   —Jennifer Kautsch
   Owner and Coach at SoberSis

"You will gain a greater insight into [the world of sobriety] and along the way learn the ABCs of sobriety."
   —JoAnne Reynolds
   CEO Sexy AF Spirits

"I related to J.W.'s persistence and positive perspective. I truly enjoyed his process and his celebration of an alcohol-free life!"
   —Tracie Hutchins
   Model and Creator and Sexy is Sober

CONTENTS

Acknowledgments 7
Part 1: Commitment 9
    Prologue 11
    Blogs 1 - 31 23
Part 2: Process 87
    A Support Network 89
    Blogs 32-74 91
Part 3: Change 187
    My Therapeutic Journey 189
    Blogs 75-101: The ABCs of Sobriety 191
Part 4: Termination 269
    Epilogue 271
Reflection 1: A Support Network 277
Reflection 2: My Therapeutic Journey 287
Resources 297
J.W.'s Core Sobriety Tips 299
About the Author 303
Reviews 305

ACKNOWLEDGMENTS

It is overwhelming to try and think of all the people I would like to acknowledge for helping me write and publish this book. I'll start with my partner L. She has been with me through my sobriety from before day one. She quit drinking before me and inspired me to follow her on a journey for which neither of us was quite ready. Nevertheless, L has been my most loyal fan and most truthful critic. Because of her, I have grown more as a person, as a writer, and as a friend than ever before. Thanks, love, for all your love and support.

Along my path, I have met and maintained some incredibly strong friendships. Some of these people I have never met in person, and I consider them to be as close as the closest in-person friend I have ever had. Carmell from Canada, Sober Sis from Texas, JoAnne from Sexy AF Spirits in Canada, Tracie from Florida, Dawn from Washington, DC, Leah Martin-Brown, the rocker from Australia, Becky Jewell from Colorado, Natalie from Missouri, Brianne Davis from Los Angeles, Brittany Priestley from Los Angeles, Bobby C. from Newport Beach, Kim from England, Sandi from Delaware, Rachel from Africa, and Megan Aronson from Arizona are all people I owe a debt of gratitude for being a part of this wonderful journey with me. Thank you all.

I have to take time to acknowledge my now eleven-year-old son X for his part in my journey as well. He was part of my inspiration and subsequently had to endure dad's absence during many hours of writing, podcasting, and interviewing. He has always been patient with me and my writing goals as well as incredibly supportive, even though he has not yet been allowed to read a word of my writing for this book.

Finally, I would like to acknowledge all the people who came before me in sobriety. While I tend to tout my sober journey as easy, it has not been easy for everyone, and to all of you, I would like to offer my sincerest regards. Those of you who struggled and still emerged victoriously, you are true warriors. You all inspired me to continue writing and to flush out my beliefs, feelings, and direction for not only my future but also the future of sobriety. It takes a village, as they say, and we are all that village.

PART 1
COMMITMENT

PART I

COMMITMENT

PROLOGUE

On January 18, 2020, I took my first steps onto the path that would forever change not only my life but the life of everyone around me. I quit drinking. Since that day, everything I thought I knew about myself has changed for the better. The person I knew for forty-eight years became a stranger to me, and I do not miss him. The ways I dealt with the world feel foreign and like a bad dream. The things that used to annoy and anger me are not worth my time anymore. The people I thought were my people, I learned, were not my people. Where once I was directionless and without goals, I became highly motivated and goal-oriented. All the time I wasted on meaningless and negative behavioral activities is now instead filled with meaningful, creative, and focused tasks. These tasks fuel my drive to succeed in the world as my new and improved self. To be honest, and this has proven to be quite controversial, my path through recovery and sobriety has been, dare I say, easy. My path leading up to sobriety, on the other hand, was definitely not.

I consider myself incredibly blessed to have been what is considered a functional alcoholic. While I do not wish the struggle of alcoholism, at any level, on anyone, I can say with incredible certainty, I was lucky in my alcoholism. I say that because even though I had developed an incredibly consistent and damaging drinking habit, I was able to get through my day-to-day life without losing my job, house, relationships, children, or suffering a severe injury. Well, at least not physically, anyway. Looking back, I do not know how I got through the days the way I did. I did not sleep much, and I was in a perpetual state of illness. I lacked patience, and my attitude toward the world and people around me was anything but positive. I don't believe I ever held a victim mentality in regard to the way my life turned out, but I did not have much positive to say about the world. I was always pretty aware most of the blame could be placed on my shoulders, and I carried that blame like a badge of honor. When I remember, which I rarely try to do these days, the words I used to use to describe myself, I shudder: broken, damaged, unworthy, undeserving, selfish, lost, etc. How did I ever make it as far as I did while actively poisoning myself on a daily basis and living in such a state of disrepair?

I went to college at the age of thirty-seven while working full-time, married, and with a child. I received my bachelor's degree and then went on to obtain my master's degree in teaching and special education. I then became a teacher and am now the department head at my current building. All of this I did while drinking heavily and in a continual hungover state.

Before I get into the absolute joys and wonder that accompanied my path through recovery and sobriety, I think it is relevant to talk a little about what got me here in the first place. If I am honest, this is my least favorite part when talking about sobriety and recovery. I prefer to concentrate on the positive aspects of making the life-changing decision to quit drinking, but I guess there is some benefit to understanding the path that leads people to addiction, too. My path began around the age of twelve; I honestly can't remember how old I was, but I believe that is pretty close.

I lived on a small farm in Oregon with my family, which consisted of my mom, dad, and two older brothers. We had two neighbors in the vicinity of our farm, but they were not very close in actual proximity. One of the neighbors was a young couple who recently had a baby. For reasons I cannot fathom to this day, they asked me to babysit for them one night. I never babysat in my life, but in comparison to bucking hay, it seemed like a pretty good alternative way of making money. So, I agreed. The night I was scheduled to babysit, some family friends were visiting from out of town, whom we had not seen for many years. I asked the son closest to my age if he wanted to accompany me while I babysat so we could at least hang out, and he agreed.

I went over to the family's house by myself to learn what they expected of me that night before asking if they minded if my friend joined me. They were fine with him joining me later. The husband showed me around the house and took me into the bedroom, where the baby was sleeping. He noted that the baby would probably sleep the entire time. Before they left, the husband offered the contents of the fridge up for my consumption, including the shelf full of beer. I remember thinking how odd it was that he would offer me, a twelve-year-old boy, a beer while I babysat his child. At the same time, I thought, *that's cool*. They left, and I am pretty sure the first thing I did was open the fridge and marvel at the amount of beer that lined the shelf of the refrigerator. I took one out, popped it open, took a drink, and probably grimaced at the taste. I can't remember my initial physical reaction to the taste, but I can't imagine I enjoyed it. I then called my friend and asked him to come over and visit.

When he showed up, I proudly offered him a beer. He and his family were highly religious and his reaction to my question is still quite clear. He was astounded by my offering. He declined, and for probably less than an hour, he sat across from me with a rigid and protective posture while I delved into the free booze readily at hand. It did not take long before my friend told me he was not comfortable with my drinking and would rather go home. I hadn't seen this family friend, whom I grew up with, for several years, yet the choice I made in that situation was to say goodbye to him and continue drinking. I continued drinking until eventually passing out on the sofa until my neighbors came home. When they arrived, it was apparent what had happened, though they said nothing. He drove me home, and I snuck up to my room and passed out in my bed.

The next morning, I threw up several times and felt like I was going to die. My older brothers picked up on what was happening and took advantage of the situation by making fun of me all morning while at church. My oldest brother kept talking about runny eggs and cigarette butts; I assume to prolong my feeling of sickness. I barely made it through church, and at breakfast afterward, I made up an excuse as to why I did not feel like eating. I somehow made it through the day without my parents ever knowing what had happened. The family I babysat for never mentioned the occurrence, and we became close friends throughout my childhood.

That was my introduction to alcohol. From that point on, I looked forward to and went out of my way to find ways to drink. I did not get a lot of opportunities at that age to access alcohol, but as I reached my high school years, I became more creative and was quite good at acquiring alcohol whenever I wanted it, which was quite often. I was a tall, fit, clean-cut athlete, and people, for whatever reason, trusted me whenever I accosted them for alcohol. People just didn't say no to me very often. I remember even going straight up to the counter and buying beer at times because I had become so confident in my ability to acquire it. Before I was sixteen, I was already developing quite a drinking habit. The second strongest memory I have of alcohol was, and I don't know how many times I did this, when I drank a glass of vodka in the shower at my mom's house before going to school dances. To be clear, I said a glass, not a shot or two or three, but a full water glass of vodka. Then, I would drive to the dance. God, forgive me for the shit I have done.

The frequency and consistency of my drinking did not deescalate through my high school years. At some point, and I have very little memories of these years, I was also introduced to marijuana and took many liberties with that as well. After high school, I joined the military, which only further escalated my drinking habits, and I will not bore you with the multitude of stupidity I engaged in while serving my country. I will say this though, because it is relevant to how I eventually found my path away from alcohol, there were times in the military where I showed up at the boat and pretended to be wasted because it was expected. I did not want to deal with the harassment that would follow if my shipmates thought I was sober. I don't believe anything else needs to be said about the military's role in my drinking habits.

As an adult, and I mean over the next thirty-six years, I continued on my trajectory of alcohol addiction with little thought of the harm I was doing to myself mentally and physically. Let's not forget the harm I was doing to everyone around me. I was married several times, though none of the divorces I would attribute to alcohol because both parties in the relationship drank too much. I drank more than my partners, most of the time. Nevertheless, I am sure it did not help in terms of our ability to communicate. As time passed in my adulthood, I began to realize that I drank to celebrate and to grieve, to party and to be alone, when I was bored and when I was busy, for every reason and for no reason; I drank because I had to.

My wife and I had begun talking about our concerns with drinking two years before we finally decided to take the fateful step into sobriety. There was no question in our minds that we drank too much; the question was whether or not we needed to give up alcohol. Neither of us wanted to accept that notion because drinking had become such an integral part of our daily and nightly routine, as well as our personal identity. During those two years of trying to come to terms with our alcoholism, we tried many different approaches to try and moderate our alcohol consumption. Looking back at this time now, it is actually quite comical. Our attempts at controlling something that was not controllable was simply gratuitous. It is amazing the steps we will go to in order to protect something we believe in, even if what we believe in is the worst thing for us. We have all done it with other aspects of our lives, too. Have you ever defended someone because you had built up a belief they could do no wrong? Then when you learn they actually did, you could not wrap your mind around the fact you were wrong? This is how I felt about alcohol. I did not want to admit this thing I believed in so strongly was not actually the friend I thought it to be. My closest and most trusted friend was actually my enemy.

In the event you are newly sober or embarking on the trending sober-curious track, let me share with you a couple of attempts I made to moderate my drinking. My go-to plan for moderate drinking was to not drink during the weekdays. I am a teacher, so it was pretty easy to justify why feeling hungover in the morning was not beneficial for my students nor me. It made me less patient, grumpy, and not as quickly able to deal with unforeseen yet inevitable problems that would occur every day. I thought, *if I don't drink during the week, then when Friday rolls around, I can drink as much as I want and not feel bad about it.* Every time I would attempt this moderate drinking strategy, I would go into it feeling like it was the best idea ever. Generally, I would make it a day or two. When Wednesday rolled around, well, there was always something really shocking, exciting, sad, and/or nothing really at all that I would use to justify why it was okay to break my moderation plan and drink that evening. Just like that, my well-thought-out and strategically planned idea fell apart; I wouldn't even try again the next day because what was the point?

Another of my ingenious plans to moderate my drinking was to never drink two days in a row. I thought, *If I don't drink every day, then the most I would drink in a week would be four out of seven days. That's a 40 to 60 percent reduction in alcohol consumption. Let's do that.* Again, I would make it a day or two, but inevitably, on one of the preceding days after a drinking day, something would happen or nothing would happen and I would find a way to justify why it was okay to break my plan and drink. Looking back at how I justified my drinking, I am astonished at my ability to convince myself to continue drinking. I went out of my way and had to even be creative at times to make up excuses why it was okay to drink. Not to throw my partner under the bus, but we both had an uncanny ability to convince the other why it was okay to break one of our moderation plans and drink. If I am truly honest, it didn't take more than a suggestion on either of our parts to get the bottles tipping in the direction we ultimately wanted them to tip, which was into our glasses.

Finally, one of my last feeble attempts at moderating my drinking was when my partner and I decided we should not be drinking at home every night. We thought, *what if we only drink when we go out? We obviously cannot do that every night so if we stick to that plan, we will definitely cut back on our drinking.* The first problem with this plan was we could, in fact, go out every night. We did this until we realized it was just too expensive to go out drinking every night. So, what is the obvious solution to that problem? We justified it was too expensive to drink out every night, so we would drink at home instead, instantly feeling better about our smart and responsible financial decision to save money. Oh, the tangled webs the alcoholic weaves in order to continue the path of their addiction.

Suffice it to say, we never found a moderation scheme that worked for us, and I am happy to save you the trouble of trying to find your own moderation schemes. If you are reading this book, sober blogs, listening to sober podcasts, or joining social media sober groups, you cannot moderate your drinking either. Skip that tiring and improbable step completely, and save yourself a lot of time, confusion, and headaches. One of the most profound statements I read about while on my sobriety journey came from Annie Grace in her book, *This Naked Mind*. She stated how most people do not drink less over time. What she means is, if you are a drinker, chances are, you are steadily drinking more over time. Even if it is an extremely slow progression, it is still progressing. For some of us, though, the progression is quite visible and fast and will eventually lead us to the point of knowing we need to make a change. I imagine that is why you are here. It was what brought me to the point of realizing I cannot moderate my drinking, and it was time to find another solution. The solution for me was to quit drinking.

After decades of trying to figure out a way to avoid the actual cessation of alcohol, my partner and I finally decided to take our first steps into sobriety. We simply had enough of the hangovers, guilt, worries about our health, arguments, the uncertainty of details from the night prior, of all the many negative aspects associated with the illustrious liquid that had taken over and ran our lives for the better part of our adult life. We had had enough, and thank God we both felt the same way at the same time. One of the best parts of my sobriety revolved around having a partner who not only understood the process of what I was doing but was fully invested and as excited as I was to finally get the alcohol monkey off our backs. It was December 2019 when we finally made the decision and set a date. We knew we didn't want to try to quit drinking during the holidays, so we picked the first Monday after the New Year's celebration to begin our sober journey. The date was January 5, 2020. Before I continue, let me backtrack a few months to better set up the events of our quit date.

In October 2019, I was already on a path of healing and trying to work through my addictions; I had several. I was seeing a therapist and had been for about a year. While in therapy, my therapist worked diligently to help me see through a cognitive behavioral therapy lens, and I fought it most of the way. I could understand what it was she was trying to teach me, but I did not know how to enact it in my own personal life. The therapy is based on the idea we develop core beliefs throughout our lives. Whether the beliefs are good or bad, they govern the way we see the world and, therefore, how we react to the world. In the event of a person developing a negative core belief, the person tends to seek out and find evidence that supports their negative core belief and, therefore, justifies it with each and every piece of evidence. The problem with the negative core belief is the person can only see the evidence that supports their belief whether or not conflicting evidence is present. Until the person allows themselves to see both sides of the evidence about their belief, they are limited in their potential for emotional growth.

My therapist drew elaborate drawings depicting how the negative beliefs and evidence fit into one another and how the opposing evidence did not fit; picture a square peg in a round hole. Nevertheless, it just didn't fully click for me until it did. I remember driving home from a session in October

2019, feeling frustrated with myself for not growing emotionally at a quicker pace. I was getting tired of talking about my addictions and not ever feeling strong enough to make the elusive steps toward walking away from the comfort that my addictions afforded me. For whatever reason, I decided I was just going to jump off the cliff and quit all my addictions at the same time and figure out a way to make it happen. I texted my therapist my plan when I got home, and I think she said something along the lines of, "Okay, sounds good." I don't really remember what she said, but I am sure she followed it up by asking me to write about the process to help me work through the feelings I was experiencing. Throughout therapy, I kept trying to use writing as a tool, but I never really found the proper motivation. I set a date and embarked on my absolutely insane plan of quitting all my addictions cold turkey.

I don't remember how long I lasted, but I remember very clearly realizing after a short period of time there was no way I was going to be able to stick to my plan. However, for the first time since I began using nicotine again, about two years prior, I had a strong desire to stick with the cessation of nicotine and give myself a break with the others. My nicotine vehicle of choice was vaping; don't ask me how that happened, it just did. Regardless, I had garnered a strength and desire to remain on the path of giving up nicotine. I told my therapist what was going on, and she was very supportive of my decision. With that, I took the first step of emotional and physical healing.

The first two months of quitting nicotine was just awful. I was grumpy and struggling emotionally and physically to get through the withdrawals and cravings accompanying the quitting of such a horrific chemical. I gained twenty pounds in two months. I swear to God, I could watch the needle on the scale move up every single day. Maintaining my weight as a forty-eight-year-old man was very important to me and had been for a long time. To see myself gaining weight by the day only fueled the anger I was already feeling from the nicotine withdrawals. I can honestly say during this time, I was doing the epitome of grinning and bearing it. I don't even remember going to therapy much during this period. I think I was simply in survival mode, and you know what, I somehow survived, barely. During all of this, and looking back at it now, I can only surmise I was sincerely a glutton for punishment. We then came up with the plan to quit drinking together. Oh yeah, that's a good plan.

Nevertheless, we set a date to begin our alcohol-free journey, which landed on January 5, 2020. We figured it would be a good time after drinking throughout the holidays and especially on New Year's Eve. For whatever reason, we thought it was a good idea to start on a Monday. When the date finally rolled around, my partner was leaving for a trip and would be gone on our first day sober together. I woke up on that day immediately regretting our decision to quit drinking and combined with my already not-so-committed relationship with nicotine cessation, it made for a very long day. By the time the evening rolled around, I knew there was no way in hell I was going to stay off alcohol with nicotine badgering my every thought, too. I called my wife that evening and told her I was not ready to quit drinking yet. Thankfully, she was very understanding, but she went ahead and began her journey without me.

The realization I was not ready to support my wife on a plan we had agreed upon together sparked a slow burn inside of me. For the next thirteen days, I pondered my plan and talked with my therapist before finally coming to the conclusion I was never fully going to be ready to quit drinking, and I just needed to take the step. One of the most notable events that took place while she was sober and I was still drinking was on a snowboarding day we shared together. At lunchtime, I went ahead and drank two beers while she had soda water, and I remember thinking how screwed up it was I was not supporting her on her journey just because I was not ready to begin mine. I think that was the turning point for me. We were planning to go on a snowboarding trip on January 17 in Colorado, so I made January 18 my new date to quit drinking and begin my journey. Since she was already traveling, my wife picked up my son from California and met me in Colorado. I drank all the way there on the plane. When I arrived, I remember stressing out because nothing was open for me to get my last drink before going to bed.

Nevertheless, on day one, I got up, and we went snowboarding all day. We met some friends for dinner, and I remember thinking how weird it was going to be not to drink at restaurants and while visiting with friends. I made it through the day and night, and the next day, I decided to carry through on something I had wanted to do for a very long time. When I woke up, I grabbed my computer and walked downstairs to the lobby, where I ordered a coffee and started a blog. I began writing a blog for day two of my sober journey. I had been wanting to get back to writing for about seven years and just couldn't muster the motivation to do so. On that day, January 19, my second day of sobriety, I vowed to write a blog entry about my sober journey every day for thirty days. As you will learn in this book, I not only wrote every day for thirty days, but I also decided to push my writing goal to 101 days and changed the title of my blog to "101 Days of Sobriety." I completed that goal and kept writing every day for around 150 days before I decided to scale back on the frequency of my blog posts, which is where I am now. I am still writing my blog, but it is now called "Sober Militia."

After I completed the first 101 Days of Sobriety blogs, I decided to take a chance and see if I could turn them into a book, which is why we are here now. I didn't think just reading 101 blogs would be very interesting, so I thought I would sprinkle in some of my history and reflections along the way. This prologue was intended to set you up with some background about me and my journey before sobriety. The rest of the book will focus on my journey since taking the first step on my incredible path of sobriety. I will pause the blogs at certain milestones throughout the first 101 days to offer more insight into what I was feeling at that time. I will also reflect on how I feel looking back at that period of my life in hindsight. There were a couple of times throughout these

101 days when I embarked on some series of posts lasting for a week or more. I will discuss why I wanted to spend more time on those topics. The last twenty-six days of the 101 days, I focused on what I called the ABCs of Sobriety, which was a fun way to wrap up the journey. I can't even begin to tell you how fast those last twenty-six days flew by. I had such a great time writing about my sobriety every day. I have kept my blog going and I have begun working on other ways to work with the sober community. I have met some really amazing people in this community, and one of the most powerful underlying themes about this whole process was when I unintentionally found the desire to be of help to others embarking on their journeys. It is my hope whether you are new to your path or a seasoned veteran, the insight presented in this book will help you maintain your focus and find ways to approach your journey with a more positive view. What you are doing for yourself, your mind, your body, and everyone around you is nothing short of amazing. Stay strong, stay healthy, stay safe, and stay sober.

BLOGS 1 - 31

Sober - Day 1

I did not write on this day because the first day always feels like an unknown, and I had not yet made the decision to begin writing every day. I began writing on Day 2.

Sober - Day 2

For as long as I can remember, alcohol has been a part of my life. I don't want to dwell too much on what brought me to the point of wanting to quit drinking, but I will offer a memory that sums up my journey here. I was a senior in high school getting ready for my prom. In order to feel able to loosen up enough to dance and try to act like I was a fun person, I had a glass of vodka (a glass, not a shot, and I have no idea from where I got it). I drank it all in the shower. Then, I drove to the dance, and I honestly can't remember if I had a good time or not.

Regardless of how I reached this point, I did. Now I have to learn how to negotiate this foreign world, this world I have never really seen without the alcoholic lens.

I have been in therapy for over a year now. I knew I suffered from several addictions (alcohol, nicotine, and a behavioral addiction too) for a very long time. I had tried the therapy route several times before. Once with some minimal success. Other times without any success. This time has been very different. I attribute the difference to the fact the person I am seeing is one of the most caring, empathetic, and patient human beings I have ever met. If you suffer from any addictions, you know the decisions you make to protect your secrets can be questionable, and they certainly tend to push away everyone close to you. I have acted in this way multiple times with my therapist, but she has consistently remained unfazed by my attempts to protect my secrets. She sees my actions and my issues as a separate "thing." Something that does not involve her, and her job is to help me see this "thing" as something I can overcome. I owe my therapist so much, and I will forever be in debt to her for her perseverance and unwillingness to allow my actions to keep me down the way they have for the better part of my life.

While my therapist has been a massive influence on my road to overcoming my demons, I still have a long way to go.

Nevertheless, it is the decision I have made, and today is day two of this new venture. Luckily, my partner is on the same path, but she quit two weeks ago. I meant to start with her, but with the challenges I was facing with quitting nicotine, I felt I was not quite ready yet. With the help of my partner, a new (sober) friend, and a book recommended to me by both, I have begun this journey with a positive feeling I have never experienced while trying to quit an addictive substance/habit. I decided to write this blog for myself in an attempt to keep myself accountable. I'm not sure how it is going to go, but I hope it will be a good tool to keep my thoughts flowing in the right direction and maybe even reach someone out there who is struggling with some aspect of addiction in their life.

Sober - Day 3

Yesterday was day two without drinking, and it was somewhat of an important day for me for several reasons.

One, the first steps of anything new are always the most challenging for me. Whether it is working out (the next thing on my list to get started), eating better, quitting something, etc., it's those first couple days of making the conscious choice to give up something I enjoy or start something that is hard that always makes me nervous. In the past, I had quit drinking for periods of time to ensure my drinking was in check. It was my way of saying I did not have a problem, but this time is obviously different. In the past, the knowledge of an end in sight made things a little easier, but it also ensured my inability to sustain abstinence from alcohol. This time, the goal is not abstinence from alcohol; it is the beginning of a new life. This is the new outlook I am trying to reframe my thinking with to achieve a better outcome.

Two, it was the first time I went snowboarding and did not have a drink for lunch. In all honesty, the midday beer after working hard in the mountains was something I craved and looked forward to from the moment I woke up. To make matters a little more interesting, my partner injured her shoulder the day before and would not accompany us on the mountain. I was with my son, but my concern was whether or not I would be able to hold myself accountable without the presence of my wife. I even talked with her about it last night, I guess, in an effort to let her and myself know I was already thinking about the possibility.

Up the mountain we went for the first run of the day. We started off the day in our favorite area on the mountain. There are several directions you can choose from, and all are covered by one lift. We had a blast speeding down the runs, looking for jumps, and weaving in and out of trees. My son has become exceptionally good at snowboarding over the past couple of years. In his first couple of years, he merely tolerated our snowboarding trips. He would have fun while doing it but never looked forward to actually going. This is the first year he has expressed a true joy in snowboarding. It makes for an amazing vacation as a family, and as a father, it makes for many proud moments doing something I love with my son.

Around noon, we began making our way back to the base for lunch and to play around in the terrain park and half pipe. I honestly can't remember if the thoughts of drinking made their way into my subconscious. I am sure I at least once thought about the difference of lunch on this day compared to the past, but it was definitely not a consuming thought.

We parked our boards and walked up to the outdoor bar and restaurant. Standing in line, I could not help but notice the abundance of alcoholic options advertised before me. I heard the hollering of people having a good time drinking and eating after an amazing day on the mountain. It was our turn to order. I walked up to the counter and ordered our food and grabbed a coke from the cooler in front of the counter. Yes, I am aware coke is not a great option, but it is something I can enjoy in the absence of the other. We took our food to a table and ate while talking about the fun we were having on the mountain. The thought of missing out or wishing I was drinking never made its way into my mind the rest of the day.

I have to say it felt really good sitting there in the middle of a mass of people with my ten-year-old son and having no urge to drink. I instead enjoyed his company, and more importantly, I enjoyed the feeling of going back up the mountain in an unaltered state. Over the past four years of snowboarding, that was the first time I snowboarded after lunch with all my faculties in place. I had a markedly better second half of the day on the mountain than I can ever remember.

I am moving into day number three, feeling encouraged and confident about the potential for the rest of my life.

Sober - Day 4

I came across a picture from my past of me holding a beer, looking quite proud. I was so proud of the picture; I used it as a profile photo for a long time. I guess I thought it made me look cool. I did not realize how it actually made me look exactly like the person I didn't want to be: addicted, lonely, unhealthy, and boring. Of course, I know that is part of the problem with any addiction. I needed to justify my actions, and I found people who helped perpetuate my feelings and addictions. I surrounded myself with like-minded people to feel less alone, when in fact, I was more alone than ever. I am beginning to realize when I seek out people and connections that don't help me, I am actually isolating myself further and ensuring I never see the other side. This has been a long-standing problem for me and one I am, for the first time, actively trying to change.

About ten years ago, I met someone who seems to be somewhat integral in my new path and desire for change. We bounced in and out of each other's lives, but now I can't help but acknowledge there is something greater here. She is one of the people who recommended the book I am reading about sobriety. It has allowed me to see what I am doing is more than just suffering through giving up something I love. It is allowing me to see that I loved something that actually made me suffer. This morning, I was having a down moment regarding one of my addictions. I haven't mentioned the third, but I accidentally began working on it this past week too, so I was feeling pretty overwhelmed. I reached out, hoping to distract myself, but it was early. I figured there was no hope to reach her. She answered my text, and we talked until it was time to get ready for work. Her presence effectively diverted my attention toward healthier thoughts and behaviors. Whether this relationship continues or not, I am extremely grateful for even the short period of time that helped me grow toward my ultimate goal of becoming a happier and healthier person. Thank you!

Tonight, I will be facing another one of those moments that will be a first without alcohol. I participate in a bowling league on Tuesday evenings. If ever there was a place for non-drinkers to avoid, this is one of them. That's not really the goal, though, is it? I don't want to have to avoid places because there is drinking present. The goal is to be able to go and do anything I want because there is no desire to drink. I know I'll eventually get there, but each one of these firsts does incite a brief feeling of uncertainty and forces me to reflect on what it is I am trying to accomplish. One idea I am trying to focus on is the fact I may actually be a better bowler without alcohol. The other, and this seems kind of obvious, but it will be nice to drive home afterward without a care in the world. I imagine many of you know exactly what I am referring to.

As I mentioned earlier, I have been seeing a therapist for the past year, working through all of my addictions. It has felt like a slow process, but when looking back at this point, I can see I have come a long way. I am actually beginning to believe I can be the person I want to be. I am very much looking forward to my next session, which is tomorrow, to talk about where I am and where I am going. Having already taken enormous steps in the direction I want to be, my sessions may have a much different feeling than in the past. Instead of focusing on why I do the things I do, I want to begin focusing on what it is I want to do now that I am beginning to free myself from these addictions.

SOBER - DAY 5

I walked into the bowling alley last night with very little hesitation or worry regarding sobriety or another first without alcohol.

I spent a little time after work reading the book my wife and friend recommended to me. It is helping me along this journey. By the time I had left for the bowling alley, I had forgotten any previous concerns I had held about the situation and environment I was about to enter. I walked up to the bar and greeted the bartender, who knows me well. She immediately reached for a pint glass with one hand and the Bodhizafa tap with the other. Bodhi had been my beer of choice for some time. I mean, I really loved it.

I said, "Oh, I am actually not having a beer tonight."

She replied, "*What*! What do you mean? I mean, are you sick? Are you trying to lose weight? Why are you not drinking?"

I am not even remotely exaggerating; that was her response. I laughed a little, then reflected for a moment on the importance of the interaction and what it meant for me long-term.

I replied, "No, I just decided to quit drinking."

Her response, "Aww, don't be a quitter." Damn!

I ended up having a non-alcoholic beer last night. I do not know if I really needed it, per se, but I thought I would give it a try. It was not bad but definitely not the same. On some level, what it helped with more was the isolation I felt in the bar full of people swimming in alcohol, pitchers of beer, tumblers of wine, shots, Jell-O shots, and many other alcoholic options. Having that bottle sitting next to me at least allowed me the comfort of not having to answer the inevitable question all night long, "What, you're not drinking tonight?" To be honest, I am still as shocked as most of them would be that that I am not drinking, so I understand the confusion my not drinking might instill. Nevertheless, I did not drink, nor did I have to answer any questions about my newfound drive for a new and better life. I also, unfortunately, did not bowl well either . . . c'est la vie.

One thing I have always stressed about when attempting to quit alcohol or nicotine was the idea of having to do it all on my own. I have tried to surround myself with people that could or were willing to help me, but when they couldn't be there, I never felt strong enough to stand up to the addiction urges on my own. This happened to me today with another addiction I am working on. I was alone, and I really wanted to connect with someone to help me get through it. I could not reach anyone, and I had a moment of panic. I felt like there was no way I could do it on my own. I sat, at that moment, contemplating what I was feeling and what the benefits of acting on the behavior would mean for me. I also considered what the benefits of not acting on the behavior would mean for me. I can't say I chose the latter consciously, but I did think about it long enough that I ran out of time and had to start getting ready for work. This may not be the best scenario for making positive choices regarding addiction, but it worked and left me feeling somewhat capable of doing it on my own if I have to. Of course, I do hope to continue to have a few people around to lean on in the dark and lonely times, but maybe I can find a way to be that person for myself at times, too.

When all is said and done, with fears, insecurities, loneliness, and uncertainty aside, I am on day five for two of my addictions and more than two months on the other. Battling three addictions at the same time may not be the most brilliant thing I have ever attempted to do, but I have to say with every day that passes successfully, I gain a small amount of confidence I can be the person I want to be. I can do the things I want to do. I am strong. And, in the words of one of my newfound friends on the same journey, "I am a badass!"

Sober - Day 6

Tomorrow is one week. It doesn't sound like a very long time, and to be completely honest, it has not felt like a long time either. A friend of mine told me this morning it is easier this time because my body has been screaming for me to stop. I just haven't been listening. Well, I hear it now, loud and clear.

It was a wonderful feeling going to see my therapist last night. We have been talking about my quitting for a year. I have been through stints without it, but I never believed it was something I could do long-term. I felt an enormous amount of pride telling her this time it was for good. I think I surprised her. How good of a feeling is it to surprise your therapist with your positive actions and behavior? It was a great session, and we talked about how to continue the idea of viewing quitting as a positive experience rather than something I am missing out on. I think that one idea is the single most important belief I could pass on to someone trying to quit. It's not a punishment. It's a fucking gift.

While two of my addictions seem to be progressing wonderfully, I still struggle with some behavioral addictions. I am incorporating some of the same beliefs and thinking with it as well, and I am standing fast. I say standing fast because that means I am standing strong but not necessarily moving forward or backward with it. I'm on day six, so I am giving myself credit for remaining on my path. I realized after my session there is one thing I really need to focus on. Reflection.

What I would most like to reflect on today is easy: the benefits of sobriety.

A few benefits have immediately surfaced since I stopped drinking. The most obvious is pride. While I may not have admitted it verbally at the time, I was drinking entirely too much. I knew it, I didn't like it, and I didn't feel good about myself for doing it. Knowing I am grabbing hold of some control of my life is incredibly powerful. I am beginning to think more highly of myself and my ability to be who I want to be.

Another benefit I have noticed is how wonderful it feels to get into a car at any time and not have to think about the best way to get home to avoid the possibility of getting pulled over. Don't get me wrong. I never drove drunk, but even a beer or two was a potential for trouble. It was especially troublesome for me since I drive a muscle car and tend to draw a lot of attention. Now, I can get into my car at any time, drive however I want, and the worst that could happen is a speeding ticket. That may sound funny to some of you, but to me, never having to worry about a DUI is an extremely good feeling. Let's face it—most of us have worried about the possibility more than one time in our life. It is a simple form of freedom.

The most important benefits I have experienced are health-related, and I will talk about both of them together. First, I have already lost five of the twenty pounds I gained from quitting nicotine. Thank God! The interesting thing is I am not consciously doing anything different. I believe not drinking simply encourages me to make healthier and smarter decisions. I desperately needed a boost in confidence, and I am hopeful the confidence will continue to grow. The second health aspect is sleep. Earlier this year, I was sleeping under four hours a night. This went on for several months, and I was beginning to panic about my ability to withstand the lack of sleep. I would generally go to bed, sleep for about three hours, and then toss and turn the rest of the night. Sometimes, I would just say screw it and get out of bed. It was miserable. Lately, I have been going to bed and sleeping until my alarm with no interruptions in sleep. Last night I slept for seven hours with 74 percent sleep quality, according to the sleep app on my smartwatch. It is the best feeling I had felt in a very long time.

There are certainly many other benefits, but for the sake of this blog length, I will limit it to those for now. Those two feel the most important at this time, anyway. While I still struggle at times with behavioral addictions, I am filled with feelings of pride, encouragement, and strength about my journey and my future.

Here's to what is to come (he says with a non-alcoholic mimosa).

SOBER - DAY 7

Holy shit! Day 7. It may not seem like a lot, but I see it like this: I have effectively made it through a week of my life without two of the vices I have used as a crutch for as long as I can remember. That's a big fucking deal.

I guess it is time to talk about the book I have been reading. I was hesitant to get too excited and brag about something until I was feeling pretty certain it was working for me. With a week under my belt, I feel confident there is a lot to the approach this book is using because it is unique and feels sustainable. The book, *This Naked Mind* by Annie Grace is an unbelievable read and forces you to take stock in many things not usually thought of when quitting an addiction. As I have stated before, it works from the mindset you are not giving up something and missing out. You are giving up something and you know you are better off. I cannot say enough how important this approach is when quitting an addiction.

I wrote yesterday about some of the benefits I have already witnessed since I have given up alcohol. I want to talk about another that punched its way into my life yesterday. Since I quit drinking alcohol, I have actually been quite busy. I was in Colorado snowboarding the first three days along with travel and taking care of my injured wife. When I returned on Tuesday, I had work during the day and bowling in the evening. On Wednesday, I had work during the day and therapy in the evening. Yesterday, I had work during the day, but nothing else planned in the evening. When I got home, I realized something amazing was happening; it occurred to me around seven o'clock in the evening. I got home from work at 3:30 p.m. and I had already made love with my wife, read two chapters of *This Naked Mind*, made dinner, and then had a sit-down dinner and discussion about what mountain we wanted to retire on.

I still had most of the evening ahead of me, and I had already accomplished more than I usually did all night. It was baffling to me. We could still watch a couple of our favorite shows on television, go to bed early, read a couple of chapters of the novel I am reading, and get a full night's sleep. What? How can this be possible? It is possible because when I went home, I did not grab a beer or a glass of wine and begin my usual routine of drinking. I did not pretend I was happy to sit in my stupor while trying to convince myself I was happy and productive while actually accomplishing nothing. I remember many nights when I drank so much I fell asleep in front of the television and barely made my way up to bed. The realization was incredible, but then something else happened—this time, not so positive.

I realized I had wasted an enormous amount of my life slowly sinking into a pool of alcoholic quicksand. That is a sobering thought.

I voiced this to my wife, and she did not have much of a response. It is simply true. We have literally thrown away time. We threw away time we can never recover; people and relationships we can never have back, intimacy with our partners, true laughter, experiences we actually remember, important intellectual discussions, happiness, love, and even tears that were warranted. All gone! How does a person make this realization and not fully beat themselves up? I can be honest in saying I do not have an answer to that question. I do know forgiveness is real, and I must find a way to forgive myself for the loss of time. I also hope those I am close to will forgive me for my part in the loss of time with them.

Please, forgive me.

Sober - Day 8

The path to the other side can be a long and lonely road, but I don't believe it has to be.

I find myself struggling to find something to write about this morning. I had a rough morning dealing with behavioral issues to the point that I was not sure if I was going to pull myself out of it successfully. Fortunately, my friend was up early and willing to chat with me, and then my partner came downstairs and probably saved me. She doesn't know that, of course (I find it difficult sometimes to be open about all of this with her because I want her to see me as a strong man). I told my friend I was discouraged. I want to make the decision to stay on track for myself, but I don't know if I could have done that this morning. I am sure we can all agree, at times, we all need someone to help us maintain our bearings. I guess this morning, I need to thank my partner and my friend for helping me remain victorious in my goal.

Thank you!

The end of the week brought with it a few more firsts for me on this journey. Of course, last night was my first Friday night without alcohol. It didn't really hit me until I was getting ready to leave work, and I had the familiar feeling of longing for the first well "deserved" drink. I put that in quotes because one of the things I am trying to focus on regarding the cessation of alcohol is that I truly am not missing out on anything. Do I deserve to poison myself at the end of a workweek; if so, what the fuck did I do wrong that week? Do I deserve to lose my faculties and risk doing something stupid? Do I deserve to say something stupid and hurt my friends? Do I deserve to risk driving when I shouldn't be? Do I deserve to ensure I will not enjoy intimacy in the evening? Do I deserve to make the beginning of a weekend start with a headache and no motivation whatsoever? If this is true, then I really need to rethink what it is I am doing during the week to deserve all of that. What I do deserve is to do what I did for this first Friday without alcohol.

It's my wife's birthday weekend, so she wants to drive up to Bellingham to meet with some high school friends. She asked if we could take the Challenger. Of course, what better way to make a dull drive more fun? Oh shit! It's been raining, and my car is filthy. I can't let new friends see my baby looking like that. So, I went home, and instead of grabbing a beer, I grabbed a hose, sponge, and soap and got to work. It seemed silly because I knew it would be raining the next day, but it was important for me that I drive my girl to meet her friends in a beautiful, clean muscle car. Would I have ever taken the time to do that while I was drinking? There is no way in hell. I would have just grabbed my beer and settled down like I always did and accomplished nothing. It is actually somewhat painful to put those things down in writing, but I think it is important to remember what I am gaining rather than what I am missing. I am gaining a life. I am gaining time. I am gaining connection. I am gaining more than I thought possible.

After washing my car, my partner (okay, I really don't like using that term all the time, so I will refer to her as L from now on) and I made a couple of mocktails. This may seem a little silly. If we want to quit, why pretend we are drinking? Well, it just feels good to hold a drink and enjoy something other than water, tea, or coffee. We then had leftovers from the past two nights of cooking at home—one more thing we are doing more of, going out less and cooking at home. It's just another benefit of this journey we have embarked on. Truthfully, the leftovers were better than most food we could have bought at a restaurant. We had a nice dinner together and afterward found we still had an abundant amount of time left in the evening. I still can't fathom the time I have wasted in my past.

We watched 28 *Days* with Sandra Bullock. I have loved this movie since it first came out. I don't know why I related to it so much. I mean, I had never quit drinking, but it has always resonated with me. It is what I call one of my "cry" movies. When I need a good cry, it is assured I will get one in by the time the movie is over. L had never seen it, and we ended up crying together. I think the most touching part of the movie is the focus on connection and how we all deserve and need it in our lives. I think sometimes we forget the importance of connection because we get so wrapped up in everything else we are doing. We need connections. A public speaker, whom I cannot remember, said something about connection I think is highly relevant to everything I am trying to do. Okay, it is not fair to use his quote and not give him credit; hold on. His name is Johann Hari. It is fitting to end this blog with his quote—what an incredible sentiment.

"The opposite of addiction is not sobriety; the opposite of addiction is connection." - Johan Hari

Sober - Day 9

I experienced another first last night. When will they end? L and I drove up to Bellingham to meet with some of her high school friends. It is her birthday weekend, and that is something she wanted to do. We drove the Challenger, which made the long drive much more fun. When we got there, her friends were meeting at a brewery. It was a nice hipster-looking brewery restaurant, but they had some amazing food for vegetarians. I don't think I have mentioned that I have been vegetarian/vegan for the past twenty years. It's a long story of how I became vegetarian and not really part of this blog, so I will spare you the details. We greeted everyone at the front of the restaurant and then eventually made our way back to our table.

The first I am speaking of was sitting down with a group of ten drinkers who were getting together to, what felt like, solely drink. The first issue as non-drinkers I can think of in this scenario is simply participating as the only people without a drink in front of them. The second issue, for me at least, was that I only knew one of the ten people. I felt a bit out of place. Both of these issues, for some of you, may seem like reasons to drink. They certainly were for me not ten days ago. However, to both L's and my surprise, we did not feel a single urge to drink during this gathering. I drank a non-alcoholic beer, and L ordered a soda water with a splash of cranberry juice. I asked the server to please bring her drink in a cocktail glass; L enjoys drinking out of nice glassware. By the time the drinks arrived, I am pretty sure nobody was the wiser whether we were drinking or not. I don't know if that was the actual intent, but it did make the interaction easier to endure without a barrage of questions about why we were not drinking. It was a win either way in my mind.

I do want to talk a little bit about what I noticed during dinner. First, L and I were the quietest of the bunch, and I am pretty sure that has not always been the case. I don't mean to say we sat there like terrified children, too afraid to say anything at the grownup table. I just mean, we talked when appropriate and definitely did not try to hijack the conversation. I think this was noticeable to me because the whole evening, I could not stop thinking about how everyone seemingly talked non-stop, and I honestly don't know if anyone really ever said anything. I simply observed, and what I observed was a testament to what we are trying to do. It's quite interesting to be the only sober people in a group of drinkers. Another noticeable observation I made was how as the evening progressed, the volume increased, and the intellect decreased exponentially. I know the idea of alcohol decreasing our intellect is nothing new to any of us, especially in a group setting, but it was interesting to experience it firsthand. What made it even more interesting was experiencing it with an underlying new belief and desire to change behavior. This certainly helped solidify some of my new beliefs.

I have mentioned this before, but what a great feeling to drive home from Bellingham late in the evening after spending time at a brewery and have no worries whatsoever about safety. We did, however, witness several inebriated drivers on the road. They made me nervous so I gave them a wide berth.

We got home late, and I was planning a trip up to Crystal Mountain for snowboarding in the morning. We watched one of our favorite shows to unwind and went to bed around 11:00 p.m. I got up at 5:00 a.m. in the hopes of leaving by 6:00 a.m. to avoid traffic and crowds. This is something I have attempted to do many times in the past but was never actually able to do it because I always woke up feeling like shit and found a reason to let myself off the hook. Today, I went to the mountain at 6:00 a.m. and I was one of the first people on the lifts. I snowboarded for about two magical hours, making ribbons in fresh powder and thoroughly enjoying myself. By the time the crowds showed up and started creating massive lines at the lift, I decided I got in enough good rides to go ahead and head home. It was a short day on the mountain, but it was incredibly satisfying. I'll be going up tomorrow too. I have the day off for L's b-day, and we are going to go up for a half-day, hopefully with a friend. It is a weekday, so it will be far less busy. I am really looking forward to it.

What is the takeaway from today's blog? I think, for me, it is simply a reminder every day is a new day with new experiences, new firsts, new realizations, new friendships, new goals, and new opportunities to create a life worth living.

Sober - Day 10

Here is a text I sent L this morning: "I feel like I could cry. I feel so much gratitude for everything that is happening."

It was so beautiful. I took a photograph from my drive to Crystal Mountain this morning. I left home at 6:30 a.m.; it is Monday, so I did not have to worry about traffic and crowds. As I was driving, I saw this straight away with no cars, snow-covered trees, snow on the side of the road, and I just felt inspired. I pulled over and snapped a shot. I took a photograph on day one of a small dirt path to nowhere, and this one was of a highway to a specific location. Can I read anything into that? Day one, I felt good, but things were uncertain; day ten, I feel like I am flying down a sober highway and already starting to plan out where I see my life going in the future. That feels drastic for such a short period of time. But it also feels incredibly realistic.

This morning was nothing short of magical. I arrived at the mountain early and ended up being the third person in line for the gondola. That meant I would be in the first gondola up the mountain for the day, and there was new snow on the ground. I have never been on the first chair. I was so excited. This is the kind of "first" I could get used to. The excitement, unfortunately, quickly turned into a feeling of overwhelming decisions. If I was to be the first one down the mountain, which run should I take? I mean, you do not want to waste an opportunity like that (I know—first-world problems). But it was true; I went over and over where I thought I should go until it was time to get out and commit. I chose the run right off the gondola and into an enormous bowl that was untouched and track-free. I took a deep breath and dropped off the edge, and began gliding down the mountain, carving ribbons all the way to the lift at the bottom. I felt like I was floating on clouds, and I was smiling from ear to ear and laughing all the way down. I have been talking about doing that since I began snowboarding. The only negative of the entire day was that L, with her hurt shoulder, was not able to accompany me on this trip. After the first run, as I rode up the lift, I texted L the above message. I was overcome with joy, gratitude, love, adrenaline, and sheer astonishment at how my day began.

On the drive home, my mind started spinning about where I saw myself in the future. In the past, I struggled to think about making big changes and about what my perfect life might look like, and about anything that was not actually occurring in the present. My therapist and I have struggled with my inability to dream. She has asked me to describe my perfect day, my perfect week, my perfect life. I sit there dumbfounded and end up with a reply like, "Why would I do that? If it isn't going to happen, why would I waste time thinking about it?" I had even incorporated that way of thinking at home when L asked me to look at a sofa she was looking at, patio furniture she was considering, art for the walls, or, on a bigger scale, a house in the mountains that she thought looked nice. My reply? "Are we ready to make that purchase now?" If she replies, "Not yet, but . . ." I was uninterested. This has not only frustrated L but my therapist, too. I never understood why. Until now.

I am becoming a *dreamer*, big time!

I am not going to get into the details of my dreams at this point, but I am beginning to see things differently. I see what I could become. I see what I could do for a living. I see how my relationship could grow. I see things I have never seen before. For so long, I allowed myself to feel scared of holding an optimistic view about anything. I felt if I got too excited about something, the letdown would be even harder if it didn't come to fruition. I may be disappointed in the future about some of these things I want to do if they don't work out, but I believe I will feel far more disappointed if I never try, and I look back on what I could have or should have done when I am too old to do anything about it.

It is time to get to work!

Sober - Day 11

First negative challenge.

Since I began this journey, life has, thankfully, treated me kind and kept stress down to a minimum. This, of course, has been beneficial for me with all the changes I have been making lately. As they say, "All good things must come to an end." I say this somewhat jovially because my journey is not ending. I am staying strong and will continue on this amazing path I have begun walking. I do, however, also say it in terms that the honeymoon is probably over, at least temporarily.

After my incredible snowboarding experience yesterday, I received a call from my lawyer regarding my ex. We are, once again, going to court. This negatively affects X (my son), as well as everyone else involved. There has been very little I can do about it except stay true to my beliefs.

In an effort not to put my son or me at risk, I will refrain from discussing details about the legal situation in which I currently find myself. I will just say principle agreements were made between my son's mother and me about the care of our son, and some of those agreements were not followed. As a result, months of arguments, miscommunications, and bad feelings ensued. We tried arbitration once, but after an agreement was finally made, the agreement was then reneged upon. Unfortunately, court became the only answer.

One of the reasons this whole scenario has been so difficult for me is because for the past four years, as a result of my ex moving my son a thousand miles away, I have been traveling down to California two to three times a month for weekends. While I truly love and appreciate the time I get to spend with my son, traveling on top of working full-time has been physically and emotionally draining, not to mention incredibly expensive. We, my son, partner and I have done our best to make the best out of a bad situation. Nevertheless, regardless of how we have tried to not dwell on the negative, the negative keeps rearing its ugly and unrelenting head.

Needless to say, having to go back to court was not the news I needed to hear in the beginning stages of sobriety. However, the first thing I noticed when I heard this news was how the information did not cause me to physically shake and emotionally spin out of control like it used to. I was pissed off. I am incredibly frustrated, but I am dealing with it, and so is L.

We recognize there is nothing we can do about the situation. We have to let our lawyer do his job, and if it does not work out in our favor, we have done nothing wrong to cause the outcome. Now, this is definitely easier said than done, but we are trying, and the most important thing about all of this . . .

We have had no desire to drink. Success!

Sober - Day 12

More challenges.

But first, I need to spend some time reflecting on all the positive things happening at this time. I am on day twelve of quitting three addictions. For nicotine, it is over three months. This is something I am extremely proud of and something not that long ago, I would have never thought possible. I no longer have to wait for the inevitable other shoe to drop because I am now holding the other shoe, and it is entirely up to me whether or not I let it drop. That is something I no longer intend to do. I am humbled and excited by the drastic changes that have occurred in such a short amount of time.

Nothing much happened yesterday of notice. I had a productive workday. L and I are not allowing the stress of the news I spoke of in the last blog to bother us. We realize it will take the course it needs to take, and there is nothing we can do to alter that fate. I went bowling again last night, no longer another first without alcohol, and it was a non-issue. All in all, it was just another day on this new journey I have embarked on.

Today, however, has brought with it more challenges. I learned today everything I have grown to understand about my job is changing. I have been in my profession for five years, and I have found every year, I learned new things and made changes accordingly to be more successful. Today, all of those experiences are about to change, yet again. As someone who relies on a structure in his work environment, this kind of change has the obvious potential to be very stressful.

While I feel the stress manifest as tension in my back and the anxiety slowly slipping into my chest, I have come to another realization I had not before thought possible. Let me explain.

I have come to be known as a passionate person when it comes to things changing, especially if I do not understand or agree with the reasoning behind the changes. I have no problem voicing my concerns when necessary if it means protecting beliefs I hold close to my heart. Sometimes, I can admit, I may overreact to news I could have been more patient trying to understand first. I am human, after all. With all this going on today, I quickly recognized I was not reacting in the ways I have in the past. I did not let my passionate beliefs overtake my actions. I felt patient; even when I was confused, I asked questions when I was unsure about reasoning, and I offered my thoughts when I felt they were warranted. While I am still the same passionate person, people have come to know me as I did not overreact. This felt really good. I have to be honest in saying, I think I like this new version of me.

There are some things I need to remember to do in times of stress. I taught scuba diving for over ten years, and there was one thing I reiterated over and over to my students. How to react to a stressful environment underwater. In scuba diving, you cannot not react; you have to approach problems with the best possible mindset; otherwise, one wrong move can mean the end. The following are the steps I taught to deal with stress underwater.

Stop: before you make any decision to do anything, stop what you are doing.

Observe: take a look around you and observe what is happening.

Make a decision: make an informed decision about what to do based on your observations.

React: then react to the problem you find yourself in.

The first step, to me, is the most important of all. If we react before anything else, I believe the chances of a positive outcome are diminished greatly. That brief, still moment of stopping everything you are doing has an enormous effect on the way our brains process the rest of the event. It allows us to make better, more informed decisions.

Today, I was able to *stop* before I reacted, and the result was wonderful.

Sober - Day 13

I've recently been told being alone is "the best." Right now, I am not so sure.

I know from my past experiences with writing and photography alone time can be quite amazing and liberating. I have done some of my best creative work while completely alone; granted, there was always alcohol involved. Nevertheless, I have enjoyed alone time throughout my life but have recently found that it is a much different experience now than in years past. Another first, if you will, on my journey to independent freedom.

I came across a photograph I took a while back that is somewhat representative of how my brain feels while spending time alone over the last couple of weeks: isolated, scared, empty, and insecure. These words are extreme words, but I feel they accurately represent what I feel when alone. With all three of my addictions, my favorite time and space to do them were during my free and alone time. I would allow myself to indulge to the point of exhaustion until I passed out, until my lungs hurt, and/or until I ran out of free time and was forced to return to life, work, and responsibility. In essence, I was numbing myself down to the point I did not have to face my own feelings, fears, or discontent.

With that said, I surprisingly feel an enormous amount of strength, confidence, and power over alcohol and nicotine. I know that may be contrary to what some of the quitting programs teach. We are supposed to be powerless, but I can't believe that anymore. I am beginning to believe we can take hold of and control our lives in terms of our actions, choices, and desires. We have a lot of power we have been programmed to believe is not ours. It comes from somewhere else. We have to give in to it in order to be independent and successful. I'm sorry, but screw that! It's time to bring independent power back to our lives and beliefs.

I'm done fucking around!

I say the above statement with a small smirk on my face because obviously, I am not where I want to be with all my addictions. The third still plagues me, especially in the mornings and during my free and alone times. I have not caved, however, and I am still holding strong with my goals, but it definitely feels like an all-out internal brawl. But hey, to my credit, I am currently standing with one hand raised above my head in triumph. I have to keep smacking my head with the palm of my hand and reminding myself of this fact when I feel like I am not acting as strongly as I would like.

I am *strong*!

I read yesterday about a therapeutic idea called "cognitive dissonance." It's the idea that when we hold two conflicting beliefs about one specific idea, we are unconsciously or consciously at war with ourselves, so to speak. This is where I find myself with my other issue, and I have not yet figured out a way to come to peace and congruence within it and myself. It literally feels like a constant battle, but as I said before, I am winning thus far. My therapist suggested I use writing to try and uncover the conflicting beliefs keeping me from finding a place of homeostasis within my mind. I have begun doing this for myself, and I feel there are some benefits to digging deeper into my soul and beliefs. Time will tell what I uncover during this new exploration of interreflection.

I am hopeful.

Sober - Day 14

Wow. I can't believe it has been two weeks addiction free. On one level, it feels like, *wow, it's only been fourteen days?* On another, it feels like, *holy shit!* Those two levels are conflicting beliefs. I have never lived this healthy, physically or mentally, in my entire adult life. If you asked me how I am feeling about my venture right now, I would say this, "I am ecstatic!" Plain and simple. That is how I feel about my mind, body, and soul right now.

I do, however, struggle with these conflicting beliefs. The first one comes from a place in which I am used to residing. It is a place of negativity, doubt, self-deprecation, low self-esteem, and feelings of worthlessness. How does a person not see the positive in fourteen days of sobriety? I mean, it's a very big deal to stay free from so many addictions for that long a period. What I have come to realize is those beliefs and feelings I have held for so long are the very reason I became addicted to everything I touched in the first place. The feeling of not being worth anything is not a good or comfortable feeling. It feels isolated, lonely, sad, and pretty much as low as a person can feel. If you don't feel you are worth anything, then you don't feel you deserve anything. If you don't feel you deserve anything, then you cannot find a way to feel positive about the outcomes of anything. You tend to go through life expecting every bad thing that happens to you, because why wouldn't that bad thing happen to you? You deserve it, right?

Fuck no!

My therapist talks a lot about the verbiage I use in my day-to-day life. Verbiage like, "And then I just do what I do (something stupid)." Or "I know myself. I cannot (or will not) be able to do that." Here's a good one: "Every time something good happens, I cannot feel happy because I know something bad is going to ruin it."

Hmmm.

There are many more but look at those statements. If I believe them, is there any possible way for any other outcome to present itself? I am virtually leaving no room for the manifestation of any other possible outcome. What makes this worse is time. I have been saying these things for so long I don't even know I am saying them anymore. My therapist smirks each time I use one. She just gives me a look, a look I now immediately understand, and then I try to reframe my statement. It is difficult to believe the extent we can train our minds to believe things that really do not have any actual merit.

Nevertheless, these feelings and beliefs leave behind enormous holes we will go to great lengths to fill by finding "something" to allow us to feel better than the feelings that created the hole. The "something" can be any number of things, but regardless of what that "something" is, it works because it masks the real feelings we are experiencing with momentary feelings of numbness. This numbness, which by definition means having no feeling, we connect with as "feeling good." If our "something" helps us feel so "good," why wouldn't we continue to go back to it over and over and over again? We do and quickly begin to forget about all the negative aspects of our addiction. We tell ourselves the bad feelings we feel as a result of our addictions are not caused by the "something;" they are the way we feel, or so we tell ourselves, effectively solidifying the belief we need our "something" even more.

And around and around we go.

If you have been reading this blog, you may have noticed some verbiage I have begun to use that is contrary to some of the negative verbiage I have stated in this blog which, subsequently, encourages my ability to change. I have said things like:

"I am dreaming, big time."

" I am *strong*."

"I'm done *fucking* around."

"I am hopeful."

"It's time to get to work."

Every one of these statements opens up the possibility for change and growth.

Sober - Day 15

Yesterday was yet another first I knew was coming but it was one I was slightly worried about in terms of how I would handle the situation. Since I quit everything, L has been home every day, so I never had to really worry about holding myself accountable without someone else present to help keep me on track. The morning alone time still plagues me with the other addiction, but that is always short-lived, and I have endured and continued to remain successful in that goal as well.

Last night was the first time I came home from work to an empty house with no plans for the evening and nobody to help hold me accountable. I was a little concerned about this, mostly because that is when I generally engaged in all the bad behaviors. So, attempting to be still and strong in that space felt a little overwhelming. I even reached out to my sober friend. I keep talking about her, so let's just call her D. I asked if she would mind checking in on me throughout the evening. She didn't respond to that text, but as usual, she came through and checked on me a couple of times throughout the night. I was doing fine, but it was nice to know someone was thinking of me and wanting to help.

I went to bed early, on a Friday night. This is so weird.

I had to get up at 4:30 a.m. to catch a flight to California to see my son, X. Nothing like starting the day off after a long hard week with an even earlier start to the day. On the way to the airport, it occurred to me today is another first; God help me. It is my first trip down south without drinking. In the past, when I arrived at the airport at 5:00 a.m., I would belly up to the bar and have a mimosa. I love seeing my son, of course, but the traveling, as well as the location, after a long week can be too much at times. So, I did what I used to always do and attempted to numb the bad feelings in an effort to make it more bearable. It never worked, but you could not have told me that back then. While I am not excited about the trip, I am excited to see X, and I believe I will actually enjoy my time down there more than in weekends past because my mind is clearer, and my attitude is focused on seeing X rather than on any bad feelings that come with this unfortunate scenario.

I mentioned location in regard to some of the things I don't like about traveling on the weekends. The location I am referring to is Newport Beach in Southern California. Originally, when my ex, S, moved my son a thousand miles away and I knew I would have to travel, I thought there were worse places to spend weekends. As it turns out, Santa Ana is one of my least favorite places on earth. Now, I know I am somewhat biased because this location correlates with traveling and that my son lives so far away from me, but that is not the only negative feeling I hold toward the place.

First of all, the entire area is just concrete. Even if you manage to get to the beaches, they are generally so crowded, the usual joy of seeing the ocean is overshadowed by the chaos of no parking, no personal space, and people generally unaware of anyone around them. I used to try and hit the beach for surfing with X on the weekends but eventually gave up. I am aware if I lived here, I might learn there are better and less crowded places to go, but in the limited time I have down there, I have not taken the time to figure that out yet.

Secondly, the need for status down there really gets under my skin. My son, at ten years old, has been obsessed with brands since he moved down there. I have never seen a child so young so completely aware of what brands people are wearing, driving, eating, and living in. I know we all use brands, it is unavoidable, but I am talking about the idea that brands actually matter to a ten-year-old. I have spent a lot of time trying to explain the concept of marketing to my son. At times, I think he gets it, but most of the time, I fear he doesn't have a clue. When he comes up for the summer, we all (including X) have a little family tradition I find to be annoying but somewhat funny as well. We call it "debranding." We try to eradicate the use of brands in the way we communicate and see the world. This works out pretty well because we just make a game out of it. By the time he goes back to California at the end of the summer, he is effectively "debranded." It takes less than one week before the first thing I hear come out of his mouth during one of our daily phone calls is directly related to some aspect of branding.

We will keep trying.

Lastly, I just don't care for the people down there. People talk about the Seattle freeze, but I would much rather deal with the chilling but real aspect of my people than the complete and utter fakeness of an area that seems to revolve around BMWs, cosmetic surgery, and keeping up with the Jones'.

Maybe that's why I enjoy snowboarding so much. The cold correlates to my people.

Sober - Day 16

Off-balance.

As it turns out, my concerns about coming down here were warranted. No, I did not cave on any of my goals or addictions. I just didn't feel as good or as strong as I have felt in the past. Feeling off-balanced this early is definitely disconcerting, and it caused me to reflect on what I am doing. More importantly, it caused me to give credit to the seriousness of what I am doing and to not take for granted how far I have come and how easily that could change if I don't acknowledge the whole process.

This is a really big deal.

I took a picture that represents how I feel about this area. Yes, there are beautiful aspects of the landscape and people, but just beyond the beauty, there lies a myriad of hidden negativities and unhealthy properties that can easily be missed if we do not look for them. The picture was of oil tankers and drilling rigs and a hazy smog lingering in the background. I am not trying to be overly negative, but the area does bring up some deep-seated feelings, and it is helpful for me to remember that when dealing with the challenges that followed me down here this weekend. One of the things I dislike about living out of a hotel room with a ten-year-old is it can get boring for both of us, but we do the best we can. We play football, go swimming/hot tubbing, and try to watch a movie or a sports event, too. As I said yesterday, we make it work.

Okay, putting the negativity aside, it is always nice to see X. We always find ways to have fun. I am so excited this year he finally seems to have been bitten by the snowboarding bug. In the past, he would tolerate and maybe even have fun with our snowboarding trips, but he never really looked forward to them. We told him he might want to find some way to enjoy them because he is going to be doing it for the next eight years either way. This year, he is actually looking forward to it. We will be heading to Salt Lake City for his mid-winter break, and he is very much looking forward to it, and so are we. He is going to start a football league for the first time in his athletic career. This, of course, is exciting to dad. He has always been more into soccer and basketball, so it is refreshing to see him get excited about the sport I love above all others. He forgot to bring his book this weekend, so I had him read football rules for youth football leagues. I know, I know, but he did it happily, though.

Today is the Super Bowl. Another first. I cannot lie; had the Seahawks made it to the Super Bowl this year, I might be sweating the no-sobriety decision. But they didn't, and consequently, it is a non-issue. It doesn't hurt that I will be 30,000 feet in the air during the game, so I don't have to worry about football parties and all that goes along with them. I recorded it to watch later. I wasn't going to watch it, but who was I kidding? I have watched the Super Bowl every year for as long as I can remember watching anything. Besides, I cannot miss Shakira's halftime show, now, can I?

I am feeling less than excited about this post. I have really enjoyed writing them throughout this journey, and I have even been excited about several of them, but this one isn't doing much for me. Sorry. As I said, I am feeling off-balance this weekend, but I did not want to get out of the habit of writing because I think it has been incredibly therapeutic for me. I have been considering how long I want to do this. I think I'll keep it going for a month and then maybe continue the sober blog once a week while I venture into some other avenues of writing. If nothing else, this has truly reinvigorated my desire to write again, and that is worth more than I can express.

Go Kansas City! (No Seahawk fan should be rooting for SF.)

Sober - Day 17

The days just keep ticking on by, successfully.

Yesterday, D sent me a quote from a book she is reading that pretty much slapped me in the face. I have thought about it several times since then, and I have even played with how I may rewrite it to better fit me and how I am feeling in all of this. It is so easy to allow ourselves to settle into our normal and comfortable living. We stop challenging ourselves; why? Do we just get tired of the rejections, critiques, and failures? Is it too much work? Whatever it is, if you look around you and all the people you know, have known, and even those you do not know, you could discern the idea of settling has become an epidemic. The quote: "But there is this: I am awake, I am alive, and I am not afraid of myself, anymore" (Laura McKowen).

When we are in the mode of settling, as I have been most of my life, we know we are alive, we are aware we are awake, on some level at least, but we are afraid of everything.

Fear!

Fear is the driving force behind everything we see in our daily lives. News stories, outbreaks, politics, advertising, romantic relationships, friendships, family, and there are many more. But think about it. Why do we do what we do in our lives of settled uniformity? We do what we do because we are afraid. We are afraid of mass shootings, diseases, political figures. We are afraid of what possessions validate us, how we need to act to keep our partners, what we need to do to make friends, how our families see us, we are afraid of ourselves.

When did we become so afraid? I am not even going to attempt to answer that question; I think that is a book in and of itself. I can, however, speak to my own personal experience on the matter. I came from a somewhat-abusive family, physically and emotionally. So, fear started for me pretty much at the same time I learned that I was fallible. If I made a bad decision, mistake, or judgment call, my father made sure I knew about it and that I remembered it through a searing pain in my backside for days. Even though I know it was traumatizing for a child, I honestly do not believe I walked through my life afraid of being whipped with a belt by anyone else, not physically, anyway. The experience was an isolated one I knew would not reoccur in my adult life. If I do not see that experience as the reason why I have walked through my life scared, then why? Why have I allowed myself to become so afraid of the world?

Why?

As a child, I think I was hard-wired to take risks. I remember finding the sport of pole vaulting interesting, so as a twelve-year-old boy, I decided to give it a try. I cut down some trees to make a pole and used branches to make a bar to jump over, and then threw a mattress on the ground to land on. It actually worked pretty well until one of my jumps took me too far to one side, and I fell on the station with nails in it and tore open my arm. I gave up tree pole-vaulting after that, but the point is, I took risks without any thought regarding the potential consequences. Did I allow my pole-vaulting failure to define me?

I don't think it was just one failure that did it.

Looking back on my life, I see the many risks I have taken, the many successes I have achieved, but I also see many failures. I believe the human psyche is programmed to remember the failures, a defense mechanism to protect ourselves from stupid actions in the future. So, as we go through life experiencing our failures, we begin to build a belief about what we are and are not capable of accomplishing. For some of us, this failure to success ratio may be very different than others. Those with a higher failure to success ratio may begin to doubt themselves sooner and with more conviction than those who see a greater success to failure ratio. I have no idea if there is any validity to this, but I do know looking back on my life, it seems I fall more in the former category. I have tried a lot and tried hard, but it has felt like I couldn't catch a break. Or . . .

Was it just my perception?

Since I have quit drinking alcohol, using nicotine, and working on my other negative behaviors, I am feeling more confident. I am seeing more successes. I am believing in myself. I am becoming the person I also thought I could be.

"I am not afraid of myself anymore."

Sober - Day 18

Yesterday, I joined the *This Naked Mind* community.

I was excited to see this group and all the people coming together to support each other to be a community of alcohol-free people. Obviously, as I have written in the past, connections are a major part of sobriety and change. As I read through some of the posts and comments on the community page, it became clear to me my experiences are not the typical experiences for a lot of people. This hit me hard and made me feel sad because as I continue to read the book, the overarching theme for quitting alcohol is the ability and willingness to not view quitting as a punishment; it is a fucking gift.

So, what is the difference between my positive experience (this time) and many others' negative experiences?

While I fear this is opening up a gigantic can of worms, I believe it is worth spending a little time on because there is a large disparity between these experiences and very little differences in the actual mechanics of what we are trying to do.

What are we trying to do?

We are attempting to recognize that alcohol is a poison and our body and mind do not function well under its influence. Then, we are trying to make the decision we no longer want or need it in our lives. This decision, to me, is where I have found the most conflicting issues regarding making a positive move away from alcohol. The decision to quit is the most conflicting because, in order to make a decision, we have to have the proper motivation to fuel our drive to carry us through our decision to quit. We can decide we want to do anything, but what is our motivation? If the proper motivation is not there, the drive quickly disintegrates and our conviction to stand by our decisions quickly fades.

Motivation.

Every single time we have made a decision to quit an addiction, we have been motivated to do so. Remember the feeling that creeps up inside like a fire burning in your soul? It's powerful and feels absolute. *I can do this. I am tired of living this way.* You may have even proclaimed your decision to others, knowing how certain you were, this time, it was for real. Remember also when you had those strong feelings, you were more than likely under the influence of alcohol (or other substances). Then, the next day, when the substances begin to leave your body and your system begins to crave them, your absolute resolve dissolves into a chaotic mess of emotional dysfunction. You no longer believed you could do it; you didn't even really care; you just knew you needed to ease the pain caused by making the decision to quit in the first place. If you don't give in, your body screams louder, and the idea of not using becomes the most miserable feeling you have ever experienced.

Let's pause at that moment.

Misery. Is there any possible way to be successful in a state of misery? This is the most valuable takeaway I found while reading *This Naked Mind*. When I quit this time, I can honestly say I never experienced that horrible first-day-off-alcohol feeling. It just never happened. Was I lucky, or was there more involved? While I feel the book helped me in a large way, there was something even more definitive at play for me.

For me, the motivation came from a deep-seated feeling I was emotionally, physically, and morally *done* with drinking.

Unfortunately, I do not know how to articulate the feeling for those of you who have not yet reached that place. It is a personal soul-deep level of angst that only allows for two options: one, give it all up and move on with your newly discovered joy of life. Or two, give in and remain stuck in the misery of feeling like you just don't have the power to quit. Those were my only two options. I knew I had to choose the first. Thankfully, there was no question or confusion associated with it this time. In the past, that was not the case.

We have to choose a better life, not to quit something. We have to see the benefits, not feel the misery. We have to believe we are strong, not tell ourselves we are weak. We have to know we deserve a better life, not deserve to feel miserable.

We have to choose to be the better version of ourselves, the original version of ourselves.

Before alcohol.

Before nicotine.

Before food.

Before sex.

Before we lost our innate sense of self-confidence and worth.

Sober - Day 19

"I love my alcohol."

I was bowling last night, and one of my team members who has been absent since I quit drinking was there. When he noticed my Heineken 0.0 percent, he commented on the fact that I was not drinking. I told him I had quit and that I am planning to stay off alcohol for good. He reluctantly said, "Oh, good for you." An uncomfortable pause. "I couldn't do that; I love my alcohol."

Perception has been at the forefront of my mind since I quit drinking. My therapist will be glad to hear this because she has been trying to jam it down my throat for a year now. Just because I believe what I feel, that does not mean what I feel is the truth. It, at the moment, is my perception of the truth, but with every belief, there are multiple perceptions that could be held by anyone at that time. It is our choice which perception we want to hold as true.

This is beginning to open up my world in ways I never thought possible.

For example, the choice of words my friend used to describe his relationship with alcohol was fascinating to me now. I say now because a month ago, I would have wholeheartedly agreed. My perception back then would have been this: alcohol makes me feel good, it helps me deal with stress, it makes bowling more fun, I need it to deal with life, I love my alcohol. But that was only my perception. As I have learned through *This Naked Mind*, none of those beliefs are actually true. They are perceptions I have built to help support the addiction I was choosing not to let go of. Those perceptions make it easier to support the idea that I do not have to give up drinking.

"I love *my* alcohol." The word "my" is what I focused on last night. The word "my" symbolizes ownership, and when we use that word in conjunction with things or people, we are suggesting they belong to us, they are important to us, they are part of what defines us. Would we ever say I love *my* pizza, or I love *my* Cheerios? No. We may say; I love *my* house, I love *my* car, I love *my* partner. While "*my* partner" still bugs me a little, the others are pretty normal. Where we live, what we drive, who we spend time with are all pretty important aspects of who we are. "I love *my* alcohol." That's actually pretty terrifying if you think about it. I know I believed it in the past. I do not any longer. Now I say:

"I love *my* freedom."

Perception. Let's say I have a bad day dealing with alcohol. I have several options, but let's talk about the two most prominent ones. One, I believe the reason for this is because I am weak. I cannot deal with life without alcohol. Alcohol will make everything better. I need alcohol. If I believe this to be true, then it is. My perception of the belief is solidified when I take a drink, or many drinks, and feel the effects on my mood, personality, and beliefs. So, I go back to drinking. Or the second option: I believe the reason for this is that I was addicted to a poisonous chemical, and my body is feeling withdrawals. I am not weak. Alcohol will not make it all better. I do not *need* alcohol. If I believe this to be true, then it, too, is true. The craving will dissolve, my resolve will increase, and I will make the better choice not to grab a drink. There is essentially no difference between the two choices other than how the choice and belief makes me feel in the end.

How we perceive something to be is not necessarily the way something is.

My perception of my relationship with alcohol is it no longer has a place in my life. So, it no longer has a place in my life.

Sober - Day 20

It would be easy to listen to all the success stories out there for people who have been alcohol-free for years and look at my meager twenty days and think, *damn, I haven't really accomplished very much.*

But that is *not* going to happen.

I feel so positive and confident about my journey right now. I sometimes want to run around town grabbing people and telling them I haven't drunk alcohol for twenty days. I haven't used nicotine in over three months. I am doing all the things I love that I forgot about because I was submerged in a haze of misery and self-deprecation. They would, of course, jump up and down with me, celebrating all my successes, and they would ask me how they too can join my path. We would start a train of people miles long, winding through the city, picking up lost and drowning souls along the way until everyone was sober and ecstatic about living the life they forgot they wanted or had.

But, that is *not* going to happen, either.

Unfortunately, while there are so many positive aspects of becoming alcohol-free, there are tribulations as well. I can honestly say the positives far outweigh the negatives, but for those who find themselves in a moment of negativity, the distance from where they are to the positive perspective I talked about yesterday seems miles and miles away. I have been reading many stories of this very situation on the TNM community page, and it makes me want to reach out and grab everyone's hand and say, "You are not alone! We are all in this together." But, of course, I cannot do that, so I reach out to people every day, offering my story in hopes one person will hear it and say, "Damn, that's exactly how I felt." Or "Hey! I can do that, too."

The truth is, choosing sobriety can be lonely.

I went home after work yesterday to an empty house; L was out of town again. My mind immediately drifted toward my third issue because there is no way in hell I am going to let my mind wander toward alcohol or nicotine again. I allowed myself to explore that place for a moment. It turned out that was a horrible idea, and it took pretty much everything I had to pull myself out of a negative trajectory and stay on my path. I even reached out to my therapist in the hopes she would ignore our agreed-upon boundaries and help me. She did not, and it was up to me, alone. As it should be. Thankfully, I found my way out. Sitting there alone, I contemplated what was going on for me at that moment. While I am sure this is no big surprise, I determined the answer was simply, I was lonely. Lonely for what, I believe, is the critical question.

Could I have met with some friends after work? Sure. But who do I know right now who is not drinking? Almost no one. I don't feel pressured or the urge to drink when I am around people who are drinking; I just accept the fact I don't like to be around people who are drinking. The conversations deteriorate quickly, I get tired of trying to ascertain the meaning behind someone's clouded rant, and I just don't feel I relate to those who need to drink anymore. It just isn't where I want to spend my time right now. I hope that doesn't sound elitist; it is certainly not the way I intend to sound. It is simply the way I am feeling about my time right now.

So, what am I lonely for and what do I do with this alone time?

I did what I used to do years ago. I took advantage of it and began laying out my next novel. I spent time organizing my writing space on the computer, I developed some characters and storylines, and I even decided on the structure I want to follow for the outline of the novel. Then, I wrote 1100 words to start my book. What? It has taken me over seven years to get this far with writing again.

Maybe loneliness does not always correlate to human connection, but a connection to our former selves.

Granted, I woke up this morning and realized what I wrote was all wrong, and I have to start it over. But hey! Who cares? I am back where I want to be. Productive and doing what I love.

I am no longer afraid to be alone!

Sober - Day 21

Soul searching.

Well, we all know it's going to happen, and today it did. I had to attend another hearing regarding my ex and all her shenanigans. I wrote about what was going on a couple of days ago. It was just a hearing because she had defaulted on a motion I filed to revisit child support based on the amount of traveling I do to see my son. The court granted our motion originally but based on her default by only a couple of days, they reversed the motion, and I am back to square one. This has been going on for over a year.

So, here I am. I walked around the parking lot, talking with L for about twenty minutes, freezing my ass off. I was really struggling, and I felt like I needed to do something, but I also knew I needed to make sure whatever I did was beneficial to my growth and sobriety. I honestly don't think I was or am feeling a desire to drink right now, but I am definitely feeling the low associated with my mood, and I wanted to find something to pick me up. So, I pulled over at a coffee shop and began writing. I figure this has been such a positive use of my time, and if ever there was a time for positivity, it is right now.

I think this is a good time for me to reflect on all the great things that are happening in my life. Let's be honest: over the past twenty-one days, my quality of life has improved dramatically. My health is better; I am sleeping more, my relationship is growing, my sex life is better, my relationship with my son is better, my career is better, I am writing again, I am considering pursuing a career based on what I love, I am working out again, I am living the life I have wanted to live. So how can one piece of news feel so damaging and detrimental to my emotional health?

Holy shit! It's perception again, isn't it?

At this moment, my perception is the news I received today has the potential to drag me down and make me feel like shit. My perception is because of that feeling, I have to worry about my goals and how to stay on my path. But is this actually true?

It is not!

Let me see if I can change my perception. When my son is having a bad day, we call it changing the channel. Let's change the channel.

I received some news today that did not feel good. In fact, it has the potential to make my life a little more difficult over the next couple of months and even years. That sucks. It doesn't feel good. But it in no way is connected to my goals or to my feelings about whether I am as strong as I was yesterday or not. In all honesty, I am stronger today than I was yesterday, and this news cannot take my joy away. I will continue to write, read, love my family and my people, do my job, and continue pursuing this incredible sober and healthy life I have recently begun living.

It is my perception today's news does not affect my overall emotional and physical health. So, it doesn't.

Back to being a "bad ass," as my friend D says!

Sober - Day 22

I was very much looking forward to getting up early and heading to Crystal Mountain this morning. It has been two weeks since I have snowboarded, and I am itching to get back out there. I woke up this morning to find the mountain was closed due to a road closure. After yesterday, I was counting on the mountain to renew my spirit and joy, which it always does, but now I guess I need to find something new to lean on for that bump in positivity.

Truth be told, I did not have too bad of a day yesterday. I felt a little down, but that can happen to anyone at any time. The difference between how I have dealt with it in the past and how other, healthy people deal with it is somewhat arbitrary if you think about it. It is simply the difference between what we put in our glass. A healthier person may choose something refreshing, light, maybe even a little decadent (calories), but we (former alcoholics) went straight for poison. That poison compounded everything from the moment we poured our first drink until the morning when we woke up feeling like death and craving another glass of that very same poison.

It's the little things.

These days, I choose a NA beer, soda water, or even a Coke Zero. It is kind of interesting when you become alcohol-free. What I consume now takes on a whole new meaning than it did in my past. I never remember really thinking about it before I quit. I just drank, and most of the time, what I drank was alcohol. In the end, I was consuming alcohol earlier and earlier in the day and more and more throughout the week. But I never really thought about it. Now it seems my liquid consumption practices are always somewhat a part of my thinking, planning, and overall experience of the day. L came home from a trip last night, and the first thing she realized was we were out of some of her favorite drinks, bad husband! It has become something we are always aware of because those fun drinks, on some level, can make the difference between an easy day and a hard day while staying alcohol-free.

Other healthy habits.

Reading and writing have become another of my coping mechanisms while strolling down my alcohol-free path. I try to read a little of *This Naked Mind* every day. I do not read a lot in one sitting, as the book suggests, but I read a chapter or two just to keep my mind focused. I have purchased *We are the Luckiest* by Laura McKowen as well, and I have already started *Rewired*. I guess they call it Quitlit, now. I like them as a way to remember why I am doing this. I have done the same thing for twenty years with my diet. I became a vegetarian twenty years ago, and every once in a while, I will read some literature or watch a documentary just to keep my goals in focus and my resolve strong. I also always have a novel close by. I love to read fiction; in fact, the above-stated books are the only non-fiction books I have read by choice in, well, maybe forever. I love getting enveloped in a good book. I love when I relate to the characters, buy into the story, and fret about the outcome. It's a wonderful way to disappear and a much healthier way than I have done it in the past.

Writing has been an elusive undertaking for me over the past six or so years. It is something I always loved, but for reasons I won't get into here, my passion was thwarted, and I fell away for a while. Thankfully, making the decision to quit drinking has reinvigorated my love for writing, and I am attempting to write every day and in different forms. This blog has been the driving force for me. I made a decision to write in this blog every day since I quit drinking. It's day twenty-two, and I am going strong. I have also been writing a separate private blog for my therapist revolving around behavioral addictions. That has not been as easy, but I am beginning to pick up momentum there, too. Finally, I have begun to write another novel. This, too, has been a little trying but I am excited about the fact I am writing again. Writing, on any level, is a step and a course in the right direction for me.

I hope to get up to the mountain tomorrow morning. They say the roads will be open. If not, we are off to Salt Lake City next weekend to snowboard with X for his mid-winter break. I really hope I can get a snowboarding day tomorrow, but if not, I have my beautiful partner with whom to spend my day.

Together, alcohol-free.

Sober - Day 23

"Live light."

Yesterday, L and I ran a bunch of errands; one of which was to Costco. When we were all done and heading out of the store, one of the cashiers said, "Live light."

What the fuck?

Could there be two words that carry more meaning and depth, especially to addicts, than these two incredibly simplistic words strung together in a fragmented sentence used as a salutation? I mean, where was this guy forty years ago when I was eight and already beginning to learn how heavily the world can sit on my shoulders? It begins at such a young age, doesn't it? The moment we realize we are fallible, the moment we realize we are not the center of the universe, the moment we realize love is actually earned, trust is something you have to work for, people lie, cheat, steal, and treat each other abhorrently at times. It happens too fucking young, but it happens, nonetheless. We forget some very simple truths about life. Truths such as our lives are our own to live, our happiness is a choice, success is a choice, love is everywhere, friendship is a gift, and we all begin as perfect human beings.

"Live light."

There are so many directions to take this statement. Here is what I found most obvious. To live lightly? I think that is a logical meaning to take away from these words. What would it mean to live lightly? Does it mean to live without the excess baggage life piles on our backs as we make our way through the challenging labyrinth of existence? Baggage such as bad decisions, negative relationships, failures, wrong perceptions, lost loves/friendships, miscommunications, ill-perceived intentions, accidents, and any other myriad of events that can add up to a massive weight we feel we are burdened with carrying. We all have it; the amount may vary, but it's still there, weighing all of us down. Close your eyes for a moment and try to visualize a world where everyone is walking around carrying their baggage as a giant weight on their backs. They have to use both hands held behind them to keep the weight from sliding down their backs and onto the ground. They have to hunch forward, take very few steps, and pause every couple of steps from exhaustion. Try to see how everyone is too distracted with their own weight they cannot see the struggle of everyone else around them carrying theirs. Try to see how, no matter how hard they try, the amount anyone can actually accomplish is minimal. Because of this, they are forced to not take on new challenges that could result in successes for fear of letting the weight fall. Now, ask yourself this question. In that world you have envisioned, is there anyone telling any of those people it is okay to drop the weight? Of course not.

Let's drop the fucking weight.

Another meaning I take from these words is to live with light or in light or as light. What is light? It is one of the most vital aspects of our ability to accomplish anything. Without light, we cannot see, we cannot make choices, we cannot perceive, we cannot do much of anything. I envision the idea of the Bodhizafa, the enlightened One, the all-seeing, all-knowing entity that is the final step before becoming a Buddha.

I am certainly not on my way to becoming a Buddha, so how can I possibly "live light" in those terms?

Maybe it just means a combination of things. To live lightly and in the light. To live with integrity, with purpose, with meaning, with love, with friendship, with laughter, and with those who make us live as better human beings. Can we do that? I think we can. I think we often do. But I think we let baggage, stress, failure, loss, and depression get in the way. All of which are choices, aren't they? Can we choose to address and acknowledge stress and failure before allowing it to consume us? Can we allow baggage to fall to the ground? Can we live more purposefully, allowing us to avoid depression? We can, but it's hard work. It's incredibly difficult to stay positive all the time, to see the good in everything, to believe we are worth it, to believe there is good in people, to trust that our positive attitude will not bite us in the ass, and to accept we have more power over our lives than anyone is telling us we have. Why is nobody telling us this? Who knows, and who cares? We just need to recognize it is not up to anyone else to tell us it is so. It is the truth.

Let's "live light!"

Sober - Day 24

Perception keeps slapping me in the face.

I've talked about a third addiction I have been dealing with, and while I have been, for the most part, successful with it, it has not been as easy and comfortable as alcohol and nicotine have been for me. Until now.

Why you ask? Perception of course.

I do not mean to continue to drive this pony into the ditch, but it keeps popping up, everywhere I look, with every decision I make, and with every session I have with my now smug and self-righteous therapist. I say that with love because she is fucking amazing. But she has been attempting to beat me over the head with this idea for over a year, and apparently, my skull is quite thick.

Perception.

What has been my perception of this addiction in the past? It has been one of no self-control, powerlessness, fear, and a complete inability to see past the addiction. I have tried to come up with external motivations to help me focus and stay on track. Motivations such as: if this, then that. Meaning, if I can stay off for a week, then I get something as a reward. Whether this would work or not, the biggest problem I encountered with establishing this plan was finding a reward I perceived as worth giving up the addiction. I came up with some ideas, but they were either unrealistic or unattainable, and this left me with worse feelings about my inability to change than before. This also led to a vicious cycle of trying to find ways to motivate myself and failing each and every time.

This is certainly counter-productive to change.

What am I doing differently in regard to perception that is helping me succeed in my third and last addiction?

It was really quite simple; however, for personal reasons, I am not going to go into details about my perceptions and actions in this regard. I will, however, speak to the idea behind the change and how it has allowed me to regain strength, confidence, and belief in myself. The change was intrinsic. Now, I know we all know intrinsic rewards are more powerful than external rewards, and my therapist, God love her, is certainly rolling her eyes at this very moment, but a person can hear something a hundred times, and if it doesn't connect, it doesn't exist. Up until now, it did not exist.

I had to dig deep into my soul, deep into my hidden thoughts, deep into my core beliefs about who I am and what I want to find the motivation I needed to actualize change. I found the motivation, but it was not exactly where I thought it would be. It was hard to *see* it because, in order to *believe* it could work, I had to feel the *importance* of the intrinsic reward. I had to *know* it was enough to keep me strong in times of weakness. I had to *feel* in the depths of my soul it was the *one* thing that was important enough to enact a new mindset.

I found the *thing*.

The very next day, I woke up, changed habits, began working out and went about my day without the behavior. I did *not* feel like I was missing anything. I did *not* feel miserable. I did *not* want that behavior in my life anymore. While I am newly conquering this addiction, I am on day twenty-four of alcohol and over three months of nicotine. If you had asked me three months ago if I would be where I am today, I would have probably laughed and said, "Yeah, that's cute." But instead:

My perception changed, and so too did my behavior.

SOBER - DAY 25

On a scale of 0–100, how would I rate my strength right now?

This was a question my therapist posed to me last night, and it was not as easy to answer as I would have thought. At this moment, I feel incredibly strong. I am battling demons that have held their evil thumbs over me for decades, and I am winning. How could I feel anything but powerful and strong? I am able to give myself credit for all I am accomplishing right now. I can honestly say I am very proud of myself and the paths I am taking. I can truthfully say I feel amazing about who I am becoming and the potential for my future. But, when asked how I honestly feel about my personal strength on a scale of 0–100, I struggled.

Why?

The question took me aback because I cannot answer the question from only one perspective (oh God help me, there it is again). I have to consider several perspectives to truthfully answer the question. There is the perspective from me as a child and the way I was raised. There is the perspective of me as a growing adult. There is the perspective of me before therapy. There is the perspective of me in therapy and the myriad of struggles that has entailed. There is the perspective of me now. And there is the perspective of me once I leave therapy (this is not an easy thought for me at the moment).

All of these perspectives offer their own data that has to be considered in order to truthfully answer the question.

Let's just look at a few. I believe the last four are the most poignant for me right now when considering how strong I feel.

Before therapy.

It is difficult to look back with perfect clarity when so many things have changed, but I will try to be as honest as I possibly can. Before I began therapy, on a scale of 0–100, I would say my gut feeling about the level of my strength was 50. On a grading scale that is failing. When I talked about it in therapy, I equated 50 to be 50 percent of the time. 50 percent of the time I felt strong and capable, and 50 percent of the time, I felt like I was incapable, unsuccessful, and undeserving. That is a pretty low percentage of the time for a person to feel like they are in control of their life, actions, and choices. When writing the first sentence of my new book (it is loosely based on my own experiences over the past year), I said, "I was a train wreck." This is not an exaggeration; I felt as though there were pieces of myself, my sanity, my job, and my relationships all in utter disarray. I did not feel strong.

During therapy.

While in therapy this past year, I vacillated between complete weakness (25) and some semblance of strength (65) over and over and over again. It has been a turbulent venture and one I almost quit on several occasions. Thankfully, my therapist had other plans for me, and so did I. There were times when I thought I was beginning to feel a rise of strength within me, but then something would come along and knock it back down. There were times when I was extremely frustrated trying to understand the process of how I was going to gain the beliefs and perceptions I needed to feel I was capable, deserving, and strong. And then, something clicked. Something made sense, and I began to think differently. I began to believe in myself. I began to trust myself.

Now.

Over the past couple of months, starting with nicotine, then alcohol, and finally the last addiction, I have begun to feel the strongest I can ever remember feeling. The accomplishments over this time have jettisoned me from feeling like a train wreck to feeling like I can do pretty much anything I set my mind to. I feel an enormous amount of pride, strength, courage, and joy. I feel like a better version of myself, or as I have said before, a version of myself before I began to smoother the life out of me with chemicals and negativity. Even with all that said, coming up with a number about how strong I feel right now was difficult. I decided on 75; here is why. I still have to take into account where I have come from in this journey. In the grand scheme of things, all my newly found perceived strength is just that, new. I do not feel I have yet set it in stone, and therefore, I know there is potential for making mistakes and backsliding from some major life event. I am human, after all. So, I feel it is in my best interest to be conservative in the number I equate to my strength. That way, I know and remember I still have a ways to go. I am on my way, but I have not arrived. I am growing, but I am not grown.

I am fallible, but I am stronger than I was before.

After therapy.

I believe with each passing day, week, month, and year, the number I assigned to my level of strength has the potential to slowly get larger. It will exponentially grow with the amount of strength and trust I feel within myself. I believe I will never actually reach 100 because I believe there is always room to grow, and as long as I continue to strive for growth, no matter how little, I will never slide backward again.

I look forward to revisiting this in the future.

SOBER - DAY 26

Productivity.

The clearest benefit I can discern from the past twenty-six days of living alcohol-free is unquestionably, productivity.

I cannot believe the difference in my life over the past four weeks. Things I have been talking about trying to do for the past year, I am doing. The amount of time I feel I have now is actually kind of unsettling. To be honest, it doesn't even really make sense to me drinking could take up that much of my time. But it did. Sometimes, I look at the clock, and it is only 7:00 p.m., and I think to myself: *I have already made and ate dinner, read three chapters in my book, wrote a blog, and wrote in my new novel. Not to mention feeding the dog, cleaning the kitchen, and putting away dishes.* I am used to taking up time with watching a movie, but lately, that seems like a waste of time.

How is this possible?

The only way I can make sense of this is to think about motivation. We have to be motivated to do things, even if they are things we love. I believe alcohol squelches our motivation to be productive. In the past, when I got home from work, the first thing I did was open a beer or pour a glass of wine. It was my way of saying, "I did it! I deserve a drink." And so that is what I did. But looking back at this behavior, I now see what followed was the catalyst for the rest of the evening. The alcohol hits my system fast, and then I begin to feel "good," and then I think I want another, and then another, and then I am on the couch looking for something to watch on the television. I remember watching multiple movies in an afternoon after work, sometimes all while drinking. I did not accomplish anything in the evenings, including spending any amount of quality time with my partner. We would eat dinner and pretty much sit in front of the television for the rest of the night.

Not a productive way to spend time.

When L is home, we now sometimes find ourselves sitting at the table with a mocktail discussing things that are happening in our lives, where we want to go for snowboarding, planning visits with X, and even just talking about how we feel regarding events happening around the world. Sometimes, we even talk for so long we forget to do some of the things we had planned on doing that evening. Of course, that never bothers us because the communication and time spent feel beyond productive. The problem, though, is realizing how much time we wasted as a couple.

It's disconcerting.

When I think about how much I am reading and writing, working on photography, and staying caught up on household chores and daily tasks, I sometimes feel mortified about the time I have wasted over the past decades. That is time I can never get back. Years of my youthfulness just gone. Quality time with my family missed. Years of creativity squandered. It takes my breath away and makes me feel a little anxious when I think about all the things I have missed. But I can't beat myself up. I am awakening and beginning to see the truth. I am becoming aware of time. I can't change anything about my past, but I can certainly change the direction of my future.

And I fully intend to.

I think the reminder of the wasted time is important. Now that I have seen and felt the benefit of ample and productive time, it would be very difficult for me to ever god back. I say this even knowing lately, things have not been going well in certain aspects of my personal life. In my past, the events taking place would have been the perfect excuse to drink and drink too much. Now, even though I feel the effects of stress, I do not feel the desire to mask it. I deal with it every day. I am still productive. I am grateful for all the positivity around me. I am dealing with life in the healthiest way possible. I am no longer stifling my life.

I am living it.

Sober - Day 27

Today is my Friday. Thank God!

It has been a trying week at work. It was not necessarily bad, but lately, it has just been difficult with some of the changes taking place and some of the new personalities presenting themselves. After work, I will make my way to the airport and jump on a plane to Salt Lake City for a weekend of snowboarding with my two favorite people, L and X. It is a much-needed trip to the snow since I have not been able to board for the last three weeks.

Unfortunately, I am not feeling inspired to write today. I'm not sure if it is the stress of work or just that I am human. Regardless, I have been writing every day for twenty-six days straight, and I have to remind myself it is okay for me to take a day off. Whatever it is, I am just not feeling it today. I am willing to bet, however, once the workday is over and I am heading out of town, my creativity will emerge, and I will be back in my happy place of reading, writing, snowboarding, photography, and family. At least, I hope that is the way this works itself out.

For now, I am going to sign off and get through the day as positive as I can and get ready for an amazing weekend. I appreciate everyone who takes the time to read this blog, and I know who most of you are; it means more than I can express. I hope you will forgive my lapse in creativity today and keep reading in the future and maybe even pass it along to others whom you think may benefit.

Until the creativity returns:

Live light!

Sober - Day 28

Technically speaking, today is a month alcohol-free.

I have been thinking about what I would like to do with this blog once I officially hit thirty days. I don't think I'll try to continue writing about my experience with living alcohol-free every day. I may do a weekly check-in about it, though. As I have seen already, and especially this week, times can get difficult, and it will be good to have a platform to voice my feelings when those experiences occur. On the contrary, the experiences I have been writing about up until now are beginning to slowly fade away, and I am beginning to see life alcohol-free as more the norm instead of the novelty it was in the beginning. This is an incredible feeling. I have noticed one aspect of the novelty that does not seem to be waning.

Alcohol is everywhere!

This is nothing new, of course, and Annie wrote about it in her book as well. As I continue to live an alcohol-free life, I cannot help but notice, more and more, just how much of an epidemic it really is.

I was talking with L last night about something I remembered learning a long time ago. This is by no means credible; it is just something I remember in regards to alcohol. I could take the time to look it up, but the reason I am mentioning it is I have not thought about it in years. The reason it came up last night is that my mind is obsessed with the idea there may be more to the alcohol epidemic than we want to believe.

What I remembered was that a long time ago, when the settlers to America began taking the land from the American Indians, one of the things they did in an effort to control them was to make sure they had plenty of alcohol. It seemed, at the time, the Indian population was highly susceptible to the effects of alcohol, which makes sense to me because I am mostly American Indian, and my entire family struggles with alcohol. The government believed alcohol made the

American Indians violent, lazy and caused them to become addicted, which made it easier for the government to take over and control more of their land. Essentially, they drugged an entire group of people with alcohol and simply took what they wanted. Again, I don't know exactly how it went down, but I know there is some truth to it.

I'm sorry, but does any of this sound familiar today?

I'm pondering how this still seems to be in full effect as I write this blog. Why else would we celebrate, on such a massive scale, something so poisonous and addicting? Why is alcohol so readily available wherever we go? Even when it is not available, it is advertised. Why are we made to feel living alcohol-free is something we have to make an excuse to do? Why do people make comments like, "Oh, don't be a quitter"? Why does an entire society of people engage in this behavior, knowing, on some level, it is not helping them? Is it simply because we cannot deal with the atrocities taking place on a social, political, and economic level? Is the goal of all the advertising to essentially create alcoholics?

It seems likely, doesn't it?

For those of you who have made the choice to live alcohol-free, what have you noticed the most about the change in your lifestyle? For me, it is the positivity, the productivity, the openness, the awareness, the idea I can do anything I want because I now have the motivation and drive I have lacked for decades.

Consider this:

Imagine an all alcohol-free society. Now, imagine a society condoning the absurdity that is the world we currently find ourselves living in. Would a motivated, free-thinking, aware, driven, and clear-headed society ever let this happen?

I am putting my money on, no.

Sober - Day 29

The world is not going to hand us sobriety on a gold platter.

L traveled all last week, so when we met in Salt Lake City, we had been dealing with our own personal daily struggles with work, life, and other external stressors. When we finally reached each other, we were so full of extrinsic negativity we struggled to remember that we are each other's person and none of what had been going on was their fault. It felt strange, awkward, wrong. It took us a few miscommunications to realize something was happening between us and we needed to take a few steps back, have a conversation, and try to figure out what was going on.

Sober communication.

We finally took a moment to stop what we were doing and find each other emotionally. While it took a few back and forths between the two of us to determine we shared the same goals, we were able to successfully do it because the lines of communication between the two of us are more open than they have ever been before. We have experienced this several times since deciding to live alcohol-free.

Trying to communicate with someone who is intoxicated, or while you are intoxicated, or while both of you are intoxicated is like, to quote the movie *Tin Cup*, "Trying to have a conversation with a fungo." That sounds funny, but in the moment of alcohol-clouded confusion , it is anything but funny. I am certain at least 75 percent of all miscommunications between L and myself over the past five years were alcohol-induced.

What a waste of time.

Looking back at our conversation yesterday, there were a few aspects of the discussion that stuck out to me as positive. One, I felt no misdirected anger. Under the influence, I remember feeling anger toward her because she did not understand me. Two, I could think. I actually took the time to listen to her speak, and then I took a moment to think about what I felt before I offered my thoughts. What? Raise your hand if you have ever spoken before you thought while under the influence (me jumping up and down with both hands raised above the head). Third, the entire time our discussion took place, I remembered she is my partner, and I love her. I remembered we are in it together, and we both have to work toward a similar goal if one is to ever be reached.

It felt so refreshing to be aware of miscommunication as it took place. I am not proud of the fact I have come to be known as a person who overreacts when things I feel passionate about are challenged. I don't believe that quality is entirely horrible, but I do believe the way I handled my passionate feelings have been at times. Unfortunately, with forty-eight years of practice acting the way I do, my behavior is not going to change as quickly as I would like it to, but at least now I see the difference. I can give myself a lot of credit for recognizing a characteristic in myself I would like to change, and now that I am alcohol-free, I have the more realistic ability to effect change in said behavior.

The door of communication is open.

I look forward to witnessing first-hand how the way I communicate with L, co-workers, bosses, friends, strangers, adversaries, and even in writing will grow as I continue to allow my mind, body, and soul to live free from poison.

Sober - Day 30

And just like that—Day 30.

It is difficult to believe and harder to imagine a little over a month ago, I was getting up on a weekend morning and drinking to start my day. I really looked forward to prosecco and grapefruit, then beer, then wine, then . . .

It feels like I have gained so much of my life back because, well, I have.

This morning, I am sitting down in the hotel lobby waiting for X and L to wake up so we can get ready to hit the slopes. I like to come down and write before they wake up because it's so quiet in the hotel at this time of day, and very few people are walking around. It gives me time to reflect and think about where and who I am. Too often, we get caught up in our daily lives those two thoughts get lost in the chaos, and we forget who and where we actually are. On day thirty of living alcohol-free, there could be no better way to express my feelings of life than with a blog about my gratitude and awareness of all the good surrounding me every day.

I am an enormously lucky man. Finding L or being found by L is one of the best things that has happened to me. She and I have found a way to work as partners like no other relationship I have ever been involved in. We all love our significant others; we all, hopefully, respect them too; and we all enjoy spending time together. But there is one truth in my relationship with L that sets our relationship apart from any other I have known. There is a willingness of both parties to fully allow—not partially, not when it's convenient, not because others are watching, but fully allow—the other to be their truest selves. Now, this is interesting because our truest selves are not always the most attractive. Imagine knowing the person you are with loves and accepts even the most annoying side of you, the most obnoxious part of you, the messy side, the lazy side, and even that weird twisted little thing you do nobody in the world knows about but them. Imagine feeling 100 percent accepted as you. I have never experienced something like this, and while it can be interesting at times, it is the freest I have ever felt in a relationship. We all deserve to be accepted and loved as who we are.

X is the coolest kid I know. He is in a tough situation with his parents living a thousand miles apart, but like his dad, he makes it work and is grateful for the tremendous amount of time we are able to spend together, given the distance apart. He is burdened with having to understand L and I have different expectations than his mom; there is nothing more important to me than his ability to grow up independent and strong. He gets annoyed with some of my expectations, but he expresses that he knows it will help him grow. He is funny, athletic, artistic, and loving. He cares a great deal about people and enjoys helping others when he can. He is beginning to love snowboarding, which is important because he is stuck hitting the mountains for the next eight years, so it behooves him to find some affinity for the sport. He loves his dad, which melts my heart at times, and he and L get along very well. He considers us all family, and he is truly beginning to understand the importance of the time we spend together. He is a great son, and I am proud as hell to be his father.

I am beginning to live the healthiest life I have lived since I was in high school. I am working out, eating healthy, not drinking, not using nicotine, and have all but lost the third issue I have referred to on occasion. Living healthy, physically and emotionally, is something for which I don't know how to properly express gratitude. I have expressed my deepest and most sincere appreciation for L and for my therapist, but who is truly responsible for the upswing in my health and well-being?

Is it me?

I am not good at taking credit or giving credit to myself for things I have done. I don't know why it has always been difficult for me. I think sometimes it's because I have come so accustomed to good things not lasting that I don't give or accept credit because I feel it won't last long anyway. What a horrific way to view the world and all the good that eventually comes our way. What would happen, as my therapist says, if I acknowledge my role in the successes I am experiencing? What would it look like for me to give myself the well-deserved credit for doing all the things I set out to do a year ago? How might I view myself differently if I acknowledge the strength, courage, positivity, and love oozing from my being now that I have done the one thing that has evaded me for decades?

What if I felt proud of myself?

I believe it would look like this: I would wake up every morning feeling good about myself. I would think about the day and all I want to accomplish. I would see L in the morning and recognize how lucky I am to have her in my life. I would think about X and look forward to every visit I have with him. I would go to work with an open mind and try my hardest to give my students the best possible access to education I can. I would read as much as I possibly can to allow myself the ability to absorb the world more fully. I would write every day. I would write another novel. I would love fully, accept new friends, be there for those who need me, smile more, laugh more, do all the things I wish I would have been doing for the past forty years.

I would do what I am now doing, alcohol-free.

Sober - Day 31

It's official—one month, no matter how you count it.

We had an amazing day on the mountain yesterday. Six inches of fresh snow blessed us overnight, and we spent the day playing in powder and having a great family day in the snow. Sometimes when I am on the mountain, I cannot get over the joy I feel from the view and the activity in which I am partaking. It is such a perfect way to spend a day off. No phones, no computers, no advertising, no television, no bullshit. Just me and my family and friends spending an active, healthy day in the mountain surrounded by clean mountain air and people who are generally in a good mood and having fun with their friends and family too and consequently making new friends.

While sitting to eat lunch together, we noticed something reaffirming our beliefs about wanting to get away from what appears to be a societal norm these days. Two children, ages five and seven, were sitting at one of the lunch benches next to us. They were obviously related, and I know siblings can be somewhat abusive toward each other, but this was just too much. The older one started pushing and prodding the younger one. The younger one started to cry, so the older one started pushing and prodding harder. Then the younger one got fed up and hit the older one. The older one thought it was funny, so he started hitting the other back. While crying, the younger one started punching the older one in the face, and the older one started punching the other back in the face. Where was the parent? Sitting right next to them, drinking a beer, staring at his phone. About the time L and I couldn't take it anymore and were about to intervene, Dad finally noticed what was happening and broke them up. His answer to their behavior? "Why don't you guys watch something on your phone?" He set up the virtual babysitter, and his kids froze still, glued to the screen, for the remainder of the lunch.

I was disturbed as a parent and even more disturbed as the inheritor of that behavior in the classroom.

L and I officially decided a while ago we will ultimately end up on a mountain. Preferably, we will end up on a mountain far enough away we can feel slightly detached from society but not so far away that L struggles with commuting for work, and I can still find a job teaching. There are a couple of reasons we have made this decision.

One reason is as we get older, we find ourselves more and more concerned with our abilities to fake our true feelings about what we see happening all around us every day. It is not that we think we are better than anyone else or that we have it all figured out; it is just that we find ourselves having less patience for things we struggle to understand. So, we figure if we find a place removed from the majority of societal norms, we can enjoy our own small little world and travel to the rest of the world by choice, rather than feeling forced to deal with it every day.

A second reason is our desire to be as close to a mountain for snowboarding as possible. We have a dream of walking to the slopes or catching a short shuttle whenever we decide to go for a ride. The view of the snow-covered mountains feeds our souls, and the feeling of the cold fresh air seems to feed our bodies. We love the idea of spending our lives in one of our favorite places on earth and doing one of our favorite activities whenever we want. Each time we visit a new mountain, we ask ourselves, *is this the place?* We have found a few places we love, but so far, it is narrowed down to at least the state of Montana, and most likely, Big Sky. Time will tell where we end up, but the time is coming.

Thirdly, we love the idea of having a destination for our friends and family to visit. Ultimately, some of our friends and family will have summer destinations to visit, and we will have a winter destination to share. How amazing would that be? This weekend, we talked about the idea of X bringing his kids to visit Grandpa and Grandma up in the mountains. The only thing cooler than that will be the fact that Grandma and Grandpa will still be shredding up the mountain with them because we have chosen a life of health and activity, free from alcohol and negativity.

Not sure why this blog went this direction, but I was not feeling any major realization from yesterday revolving around living alcohol-free. Although, it could be argued living this way is opening my mind more and more to the possibilities of living any life I choose. If that is the case, the above is what I choose, and it is truly my hope to be a couple that the young kids point at as we jump, shred, and ride down the mountain with gray hair and out-of-date gear and say: "I want to be like that couple when I am older."

PART 2
PROCESS

A SUPPORT NETWORK

One of the things you will begin to see throughout my blogs and especially in my reflections is the overarching theme that sobriety does not have to be hard. I know that is a very controversial topic and one for which I have received some backlash, but I have to stay strong in my beliefs. I believe, given the right circumstances, sobriety can actually be quite easy. With this in mind, I decided to use these reflection moments throughout my book of blogs to talk about the most poignant aspects of my sobriety that led me to belief sobriety is, in fact, easy.

There is no question a positive support network is necessary for everyone, but for addicts, it is essential. While many people tend to think of sobriety as lonely, I believe active addiction is even lonelier. Because of this, we, as addicts, tend to isolate ourselves, even in the company of others, and we get used to dealing with life on our own. The shift from active addiction into recovery can be a lonely one, so it is imperative we find people who either understand what we are going through or people who can at least relate to what we are going through on some level. Sometimes, our support network can make the difference between successful or failed sobriety.

You will find the extended reflection on the importance of a support network on page 277.

BLOGS 32-74

Sober - Day 32

The first month passed with minimal issues, and I am incredibly proud I was able to stick to my goal of writing about my experience every day for thirty-one days. I would have to say it was one of the most therapeutic tools I could have used, and I would recommend it to anyone who is attempting to take on something that feels overwhelming or bigger than themselves. For me, it was something I *had* to do every morning, and my belief of having to get it done kept me focused on my path throughout the rest of my day.

I mentioned earlier in my blogs about what I would do with my writing after the first full month was over. I have decided to take it in another direction. I am still going to use this medium as a way to express my experiences when things get difficult, which I honestly don't foresee too much of at this point, but I know things can change and happen that we do not expect. I will write about them when they do. I am also going to begin including some photography into the mix. I have been thinking about trying to force myself to get out there and photograph more and then write about what I capture. I am not sure how this is going to work yet, but I think it could be a great way to keep me writing and taking photographs.

I have also created a lofty goal for myself in a bigger vein. As I have mentioned earlier, I have begun writing another novel. I have decided to have a finished first draft of my manuscript by my birthday, April 30. This requires me to write about 1,200 words a day. This is not too difficult for me once I get rolling, but it will make keeping the sober blog moving at full speed difficult. So, I will write when I feel inspired by a specific journey or when a photograph inspires me to write, but the rest of my energy for the next two and a half months will be on my novel. Once completed, I am considering taking it to a writing conference to see if I can find any interest. I tend to work better under deadlines and goals, so here we go.

This is a big one.

At the very least, I will write once a week for my sober blog; it has been such a helpful activity for me. I will miss the daily drive to post, but hopefully, I can redirect that drive into my novel.

One of my favorite discoveries over the past thirty-two days has been the quote from the Costco guy. "Live light!"

Off I go, living light and loving life as a new man on a new journey with endless possibilities.

Sober - Day 33

What is with the sober hangovers?

Just when I feel I am ready to let go of the daily writing about my experiences alcohol-free, I wake up and feel like I had an epic night of tying one on.

Of course, this is not the case.

If I'm honest, I guess I know what is going on for me, and it has nothing to do with living alcohol-free or whether or not I am ready to tackle life without this blog. It is the fact that I am struggling a little in my professional life. A week or so ago, I spoke briefly about changes occurring at my workplace and how I did not feel great about the changes. I went into the changes with an open mind and was trying to find ways to make it work within the construct of what they were asking, but I am just not seeing it.

I am in my fifth year at my job, and it took me this long to get to a place where I could say I felt like I was good at my job and I was making positive progress. I am not where I want to be, mind you, but I am moving forward and feeling good about what I am doing. These changes have put me back to feeling like I am starting over, and I do not feel confident in how my supervisors view me and my performance. This is not a good feeling for me.

With that in mind and the fact that my son is visiting for the whole week for his mid-winter break while I am at work is not helping my outlook at the moment either. It is hard enough to be away from him, and generally, we have the same time off, so when I have him, I am not working. But this time, that is not the case, and I am feeling the disconnect combined with my unease at work.

Needless to say, you can probably discern why I am feeling a need to write this morning rather than taking the break I said I would. I just thought it would be therapeutic for me to get some thoughts out and see if it helps to set my mind at ease. I believe it is helping already because I am able to see that even though things feel heavy and I don't like the way I feel, all of these disturbances are situational and manageable. I can take a step away from the negative feelings and concentrate on the positives.

I successfully wrote in my novel yesterday for my goal of having a completed rough draft by my birthday, which felt good. I went bowling and spent another night surrounded by people drinking, and I did not feel even a twinge of a desire to drink. I have an amazing partner, an incredible son, a great home, an awesome car, and I am beginning to build some friendships that are more positive than I have experienced in a long time.

Life is pretty fucking outstanding, actually. Okay, on with the day! Thanks for reading.

SOBER - DAY 34

I had a productive session with my therapist last night. As I continue to check things off my list of behaviors I want to change, I am quickly coming to the realization my time in therapy is coming to an end. While this is the ultimate point and goal, it also comes with a certain amount of sadness for me. You see, I have been seeing a therapist for over a year now, and in that time, I have gone through some difficult growing pains in my journey to emotional and physical freedom. I have had to admit a lot of uncomfortable things about myself. I have had to acknowledge some truths that were counter-intuitive to my personal perceptions before I began all of this. I have had to learn how to deal with life, stress, hardships, joy, happiness, and every other emotion known to mankind without the addition of the external chemicals and influences that have been a part of my life for decades. All of these things I have done with the presence of another human being who sat with me through it all. There is no way not to feel a certain amount of attachment to someone in such a setting. So, with boundaries and professionalism aside, I am going to be losing a close friend very soon.

The interesting part of this friendship is it is essentially one-sided. The therapist certainly has an emotional investment in their client to some extent, but the investment is, for the most part, clinical. For the client, the investment comes in the form of trust, friendship, admiration, mentorship, and acceptance. When you think about the human psyche and how it works within the human condition, people are really not built to withstand this kind of loss, clinical or personal. With that said, and regardless of how I feel about it, this loss is coming, and I have to consider what it will mean for me and my future.

When asked by my therapist how I feel about the imminent loss, my response was, with slight trepidation, I will be fine. Of course, I will be fine, but it does not mean I am happy about it. Last night, L acknowledged some feelings of unease about my time in therapy and, more specifically, about my feelings toward my therapy and therapist. I cannot argue with or hope to change these feelings for her, but I hope the overall takeaway from this experience is one of incredible growth and appreciation for what has come from my time with my therapist in therapy.

The bigger question for me, at this point, is what will life look like after therapy?

The honest truth of the matter is that it will not be much different. I am still living my life and making decisions on my own that have been positively benefiting my growth and, therefore, my life. All of these decisions and changes in mindset have ultimately been made by me; whether another person was present in the guiding of these changes or not, they were mine. I own them. I have grown, and I have changed my perceptions of who I am and for what I am capable of. On some level, I believe there is a small amount of discomfort for me in taking all the credit when I know there was someone else whose presence was invaluable in my growth, but I am working on accepting that as well.

I need to build up my circle of friends as I move further into this new life I have built for myself. I have an amazing partner who is ultra-supportive of me and everything I am attempting to accomplish. We are truly partners and can rely on each other for anything. I am working on building some friendships, too, that I hope will be mutually beneficial. I find friendships have always been somewhat difficult for me. I am not exactly sure why this is true, but I know I have struggled with them in the past. Sometimes, I feel it is a trust issue. I have a hard time trusting people because I feel I have been burnt too many times. Other times, I feel it is more to do with the fact that I don't meet a lot of people I want to be friends with, so when I do, I tend to go all-in and probably come across as somewhat suffocating to people. Either way, these are both aspects of my personality I can work on moving forward.

This evening, L and I are having some new friends over for dinner. They have a ten and eight-year-old, and X is here, so it will be fun to see how they get along. We are excited to spend some time with our new friends, too, so it is kind of a double playdate. I guess we will see how it goes. We are doing a taco night, so I had to let them know L and I are not drinking in case they wanted to bring their own libations. She said her husband doesn't drink much anyway, and she is going to take the night off, so that already seems to be working out well. It will be our first get-together at home with people outside of the book club since we quit drinking. I am looking forward to it.

Here's to new friends and relationships and to the eventual loss of old ones.

Sober - Day 35

TGIF! Truly.

It's been a trying week for me, and I am ready for the weekend. L, X, and I have been enjoying our time together, but I have been tired from work and not as present as I would like to be with X. Last night, our friends were not able to come over, but it worked out well because we all just had a mellow night together. We made tacos, watched a movie, and I fell asleep on the sofa while L and X watched a show together.

Today, immediately after work, we are heading up to Crystal Mountain for snowboarding. I can't think of a better way to wrap up the week than doing something healthy, in nature, and with my favorite people. It will be a much-needed day of fun, and I cannot wait.

In terms of living alcohol-free, I would say the lows are quite different these days. Living without alcohol does not negate hard days, difficult situations, bad feelings, or even anger. It does, however, negate the *need* for something (external) to fix it. What I am noticing very quickly is how I am handling these unwanted yet natural feelings. In fact, I may go so far as to say I am noticing how I am *not* really *handling* these unwanted feelings at all anymore. They are becoming normalized, and by normalized, I mean they are beginning to feel like any other feeling I have on a daily basis. I have never felt the need to suppress the feeling of being tired or curious, happy, or any other mundane events of daily life.

So, why are negative feelings so deserving of suppression?

Could it be as simple as perspective, yet again? I believe it is. Now, with all that is going on in my world I could define as negative, unwanted, or anxiety-producing, I am no longer feeling a need to suppress those feelings. Other than taking the time to write about them, I am starting to think that I am beginning to see no differentiation between them and what I would call positive feelings.

They are just feelings.

I feel them, sit with them, try to understand their origins and purpose, do my best to make emotionally sound decisions regarding them, and then move the fuck on.

I am no longer feeling those negative feelings and thinking to myself, *damn! I cannot handle these feelings*. I do not think the only way I can get through a negative situation is to drown it in a pool of poison in a feeble attempt to make it temporarily disappear and pretend like it doesn't exist. I am definitely not waking up the next day and feeling the need to do it all over again. I am not so disillusioned I actually thought my problems ever disappeared when I drank. I am not clueless to the fact my impending hangover is going to make me less motivated, grumpier, and less likely to be able to actually deal with the problem I attempted to suppress in the first place.

No, I am definitely not doing that.

My perspective is changing, and it looks more like this. Negative feelings are just feelings, and they are only negative because I give them power. The moment I decide they are no longer negative is the moment they become the mundane, just another simple notion that crosses my daily path and I work through with very little thought or energy expended because I am now aware.

I read the following recently, and I think it fits this blog post:

"We are what we think. All that we are arises with our thoughts" (Buddha).

Sober - Day 36

I had a magical Friday night, and there was no alcohol involved.

Immediately after work, we headed up to Crystal Mountain for some nighttime snowboarding. I have not done a lot of night boarding, so this was new for all of us. It was a clear night and relatively warm and quite beautiful. I cannot think of a better way to spend the end of a week than with the people I love and doing something that brings us so much peace. We all laughed, played, and had an amazing time. Even my ten-year-old was filled with joy and appreciation for the time spent together in such a healthy environment. Afterward, we went out for a nice dinner with live music and then headed home tired and ready for a good night's sleep.

I slept for nine hours. I haven't slept that long in a decade.

This morning I woke with the sober-hangover feeling, I am assuming from dehydration, but I also think from sleeping for so long. My body had no idea what to do with that much sleep. While sipping my coffee and trying to allow my body to slowly reinvent itself, I had an interesting conversation with L. You know, those conversations that are meaningful, reciprocal, and interesting. The conversations we long forgot we could have while we were drinking every day. During our conversation, the idea of whether or not it is a good idea to believe having a celebratory drink for a special occasion is suitable or not. L believes she will be able to do that in the future, which is fine for her because we definitely had different demons in terms of alcohol. She could drink during the day and still accomplish more in a day's time than most people can in a week. For me, if I started drinking, my day was done.

The conversation got my mind spinning.

We all know everyone has different reactions to alcohol. We have our own demons affecting us differently, and we all have different ways of trying to manage those demons. I have always been aware of what my demons looked like, but since I have quit drinking, I have begun to recognize those demons in an even clearer light. For me, once I made the choice to have a drink, I could pretty much write off getting anything productive done that day. Even worse than that, once I had a drink, I believe a chain reaction took place lasting anywhere from a short period to several days to a week or more. It went like this: I would have a drink, let's say, on Saturday morning to celebrate the weekend. After that, more drinks would follow, and then I would only want to engage in things that suited drinking, like watching television, a movie, or anything that really didn't require much energy, mentally or physically. The day and evening would follow in a similar vein until I eventually fell asleep, usually on the couch. I never really passed out from drinking, but I did drink until I slowly drifted off to sleep. The next day, I would wake up with a hangover and, of course, cure it by having a mimosa, and the whole ordeal would repeat itself. That was a vicious cycle and one from which it became increasingly difficult to break away. The cycle occurred during the week, too. No, I would not drink in the morning during the week, but I would think about my ensuing first drink all day long until it was time to enjoy the first libation and once again begin the cycle over and over again.

The point is this. Once the cycle begins, all productivity stops, and I can pretty much write off any productivity for my life. It's literally like throwing away days of my life each time I choose to take a drink. That sounds a little harsh, but is there truth to it? I believe there is, and the more I consider all the time I have lost, the more I believe the following:

No, it is not suitable for me to drink alcohol on any occasion anymore.

We are staying in a hotel in the city tonight. One of our favorite artists, ZZ Ward, is playing at the Showbox. This will once again be a first without alcohol. You know what I am thinking about as I get ready to head to a live concert without alcohol? How much more I will remember from the evening and how much more fun I will have attending something I love with mental clarity and presence of mind. I think it may be an interesting realization. In the past, I have always equated my favorite things with drinking and sometimes barely remember what actually took place while doing something I love.

Here is to a fun night out with L and to a fun night to *remember*.

Sober - Day 37

There is so much happening right now.

Last night was a wonderful night out with L. ZZ Ward put on a spectacular show, and more importantly, I remember every single detail of the experience. It was uncanny how, after writing about not remembering things from our drinking days, on the way to the concert, I could not recall where I last saw ZZ perform. It made me laugh and even more thankful for what I am doing with my life. L is having very similar feelings and experiences, and we love sharing them with each other as they surface.

I do wonder, however, if you ever really get used to the way people act and behave while drinking out in public when you are sober. I had to remind myself on several occasions that a particular person who was annoying me was probably me not very long ago, and I needed to give them a break. On some level, it's actually quite embarrassing to witness the lack of awareness, the absence of personal space, the overbearing volume of voices, the shallowness of conversations, and even the simple smell of inebriation. It is so incredibly noticeable now.

Don't get me wrong.

I am certainly not trying to pat myself on the back as if to say I am some enlightened being who is above everyone else. Anyone who knows me knows this is far from how I feel about myself. Although, that is beginning to change as I learn more about my potential throughout this journey. Even still, I do not think I am better than anyone else. I just can't help but notice the absurdities present, accepted, and even encouraged with the societal norm of intoxication. I imagine anyone who has quit drinking knows exactly what I am referring to, and anyone who has not thinks I am a self-righteous asshole. Fortunately, I am fine with either. I am beginning to care less and less about what people think of me and to be honest, it's about fucking time.

Something else happened to me this morning that I was utterly not prepared for. I began reading another Quitlit book called *We Are the Luckiest* by Laura McKowen. I did not get through the introduction before I had a full-blown mental meltdown in bed right beside L. I threw the book I was reading down, tossed my glasses on the bed, and began crying my eyes out. Of course, since I do not allow myself to cry over real things, I held back as many of the tears as I could but still managed to squeeze out a few. L was blown away; she had never seen me react in such a way to anything.

What hit me so hard?

It really wasn't that big of a deal. To anybody else, the passage I read would not affect them in the same way. It was not emotionally touching; it did not carry a ton of spiritual weight; it was not an enlightening realization about why we are on this planet; it wasn't really much of anything to most people. To me, though, I read words from another human being that mirrored my own feelings about who I am, what I have been through, where I want to go, and where I am actually going. I heard myself speaking through the words of another person who has experienced my life and is now living a life they are proud of, that they want to share with others, and that they know they deserve. It hit me so incredibly hard because reading those words from Laura McKowen meant I no longer have an excuse not to succeed. I no longer have an excuse to be anything but exactly the man I want to be. I no longer have an excuse to do anything other than everything I want to do with my life.

I am free to be the man I always dreamed I could be.

Sober - Day 38

Back to work after an incredible weekend.

I completed all my goals for the weekend, stayed on my sober path, but I am in no way ready to go back to work. Nevertheless, Monday is here, so I might as well make it as good a day as possible. I was hoping to ride my bike this morning, but I couldn't quite pull it together, so I will make sure to get a ride in before counseling tonight. L is gone for the week, so I plan on focusing on the writing of my novel and reading. I absolutely love the way I spend my evenings these days. Productive.

With all honesty, I am not feeling a whole lot of new creativity flowing through me this morning, so I think I will just keep it short and say I did my check-in for the blog and forgive myself for not writing something inspiring or interesting. Sometimes, I think it is okay to just be present and not worry about all the things happening for me throughout this journey.

Today, I think I will just focus on all the positive things happening in my life, all the wonderfully supportive people around me, all the new friends coming my way, all the new adventures waiting to be had, and all the love that seems to be swirling around me now that I can actually accept it.

I will also put out into the universe my positive energy for anyone struggling with addiction, life, work, relationships, creativity, or just decisions. I hope everyone has a wonderful day and finds love, creativity, and support whenever you need it.

"Live light."

Sober - Day 39

I ended up having a low moment yesterday.

We know they are coming and we are only human, but sometimes, I feel like things are going so well I should be able to handle all the human distractions. But I am not quite there yet, and I must acknowledge there will be good, bad, great, and even terrible days, and that is okay.

I went to therapy last night, and I was feeling a little low, not down, just a little low of energy. We talked through a couple of things that were going on for me, and then the conversation slowly shifted to talking about goals. I talked about all the things I want to do and how I am able to set goals and actually see them coming through fruition. Once the conversation began, I felt like a completely different person. I felt light and energetic. I felt the concerns of the day slide down and away from me. I felt positive, and I felt noticeably happier.

Why?

Nothing changed. The day had still happened. Whatever caused my energy to sink lower than I was comfortable with still occurred. I had made no visual changes to anything around me. I had only changed one thing. You will be surprised to know it's not perception this time, though it could be argued perception played a big role here too. This time, I am thinking about focus. My focus changed. Perception is how we view certain events. How we feel about what happened, what we could have done differently, what good we can find, and what negativity we can let go of. All of these things stem from our vantage point. But the focus, now focus, is a shift in our views wholly. It's like watching a movie on the back of your seat during a flight. If you turn your head and begin watching a different movie on somebody else's screen, your mind has to let go of everything it was taking in from your movie to take in what is happening in the new movie. You can't carry the events of your movie with you and apply them to the events happening in another movie; they will not correlate.

So, when I began talking about my goals and all the good and positive things happening in my life, I did not have to consciously let go of the negative things I was feeling. The positive just overtook the negative, and I was left feeling nothing but what the positive feelings brought with them.

Why wouldn't we just walk around thinking positive thoughts all day long?

I believe our bodies and minds are made to prepare for and endure battle. We are hardwired to deal with conflict from back in the days when survival may not have been a given. When we had to fight and struggle for every meal, when sleeping was not safe, and when procreation was a necessity. During these times, our minds and bodies had to be ready for anything and everything negative that could potentially happen. We were constantly on guard for our lives. With that in mind, it would make sense for our mindset to lean toward what could go wrong or how we need to protect ourselves from harm. Today, we do not live in such a world. It may feel like it sometimes, but let's be honest, we don't. We do not have to think about worst-case scenarios anymore, but we are still hardwired to do so.

What is easier for our minds and bodies to accept? Positive thoughts or negative thoughts?

I think we are built to think negatively, which means, in order for us to live in a world of positivity, we have to consciously make a choice to think in a positive way every single day. It does not come naturally. That is a heavy burden if you think about it. If it is easier for us to be in fight-or-flight mode all the time, why would we choose the more difficult road?

Because it's awesome.

It feels so good to feel positive, to be productive, and to find joy in more things. Our world opens up, and we see things we never knew existed. It reminds me of a conversation I recently had with my son about food. I try to explain to him if he chooses to like healthier foods, he will and how much more fun will the world be if he enjoys more of his meals? Doesn't the same thing apply to us adults and the way we choose to live our lives?

If we choose to enjoy more things, how much more fun will our world be if we are constantly finding joy in everything we do?

Sober - Day 40

Forty days and forty nights, alcohol-free.

And so he set out on his lonesome journey for forty days and for forty nights, knowing the devil would follow in every impression his feet made into the earth. He knew the path was long and he would be tempted at every turn, down every straight away, and even when he wasn't moving. It would be up to him to stand up against the evils that stood as obstacles between him and his goal. He could give in, take the easy path and let the negative energy overtake his spirit and live among the masses, or he could be strong, fight each and every temptation like it was the last thing standing before him and his personal quest for a better life. Because let's be honest, at this point, each temptation may be his last chance for survival. And so he fought day and night, trudging through the forest of lies and misconceptions, keeping his eyes on the truth he is slowly beginning to unveil. Each passing day is another day the devil can't have back, and this fuels his determination to keep fighting because he knows now he can beat the devil by not listening to or giving credit to his deceptions. The devil eventually becomes weakened, and in seeing this, the warrior becomes even stronger until on the fortieth day, he emerges from the depths of hell with his head held high and his confidence pouring through his heart and soul, and he says, "You cannot keep me down by drowning my spirit with your evil libations. I see you, I know the truth, and I will spread the word of your treachery until every last person agrees to stand up and fight you to the death."

Okay, just give me that. I was in a mood this morning.

I do not consider myself a religious person; however, if there is significance to the above saying, I'll jump on the bandwagon and say I have made it through forty days and forty nights of living alcohol-free and scream "Hallelujah" at the top of my lungs to anyone who cares to hear. You want to know why?

Because I fucking deserve it. And so does anyone who sets out to conquer a demon, and even after many failed attempts, they continue to fight until eventually slaying whatever evil that has kept them down and away from their dreams. I'm not going to lie; I feel like a warrior right now. I feel as though I have been to battle and returned victoriously. I am smart enough to know my battling days are far from over, but this one, this particular one on this fortieth day, I have emerged with my hands raised above my head, and I feel more alive and confident than I may ever have felt in my entire life. That is worth celebrating.

Maybe the whole thirty days of sobriety thing needs to be changed to forty days and forty nights since there is an age-old mystique to this length of time, whether it has any merit or not. I kind of like the sound of it, anyway. That's why I wrote the first paragraph the way I did; I just had a feeling, and I wanted to explore the feeling for a moment. I was going to erase it and start over, but I thought, *what the hell*; the point of this blog is to explore some of my feelings and experiment with how I am dealing with life throughout this journey.

So, there you go. I apologize if it was a little over the top for some of you, but it was kind of fun for me, nonetheless.

To all my fellow warriors, go forth and conquer your demons not one day at a time, but one life at a time, and fear not, for you are not alone in your journey; you have many fellow warriors among you who need only your desire to reach out for us to come running to lend a hand in your fight for victory over our common enemy.

SOBER - DAY 41

Alcohol-free or sober does not mean *we* have a "problem."

It means we have recognized *alcohol* is a problem, and we have allowed it to control us for far too long, and we no longer want it to be a part of our lives. I have read about this in Annie Grace's book *This Naked Mind* and other literature. It never really hit me as a true thing until recently. I have been paying a little closer attention to the way the media spins the idea of not drinking alcohol.

I watch television shows while I work out on my bicycle. Today, while watching one of my guilty pleasures, the topic of sobriety came up in the story. A woman was talking with one of her new friends who came over to visit and brought a bottle of wine. The new friend asks if she is ready for a glass, and the sober woman says, in a very subdued somber voice, "I can't. I'm actually sober." The new friend's face sinks, and she looks as though she is talking with someone who just lost a loved one. She pauses for a moment and then says, "I'm so sorry, I didn't know; that must be really hard." She then places a consoling hand on the sober friend's shoulder. The sober friend subsequently looks down at the floor with slumped shoulders and says, "Yes, it is. But I'm getting better every day."

What the fuck?

No wonder quitting alcohol is so stressful for people. It is not the alcohol that makes it difficult; it's the stereotypical belief about sobriety and the stipulations placed on those who choose not to drink. We are outcasts; they may as well throw us in a colony on some island like they did for people with leprosy. Is it contagious? What if I want to quit drinking, too? We can't allow that. Get rid of them. I realize this is an over-dramatization but is it really? I know I prepare myself for what I am going to say anytime I walk into a new situation where drinking will be involved and I will not be partaking.

I wonder if people who never drank experience any of these feelings. There is a social experiment for you. Do people who never have drunk alcohol feel the looking-down-the-nose from others when they say they don't drink? Or is this lovely pastime just reserved for us ex-addicts? Do they somehow know we used to drink and now we don't, so they assume there must be something wrong with us? Are we just aware that for a long period of time, we were controlled by something we no longer find attractive and are more aware of those who still see the attraction, so their reactions are more pronounced? I don't know what it is, but it is something, and it is a valid concern for anyone wanting to live alcohol-free.

It has been nice finding the TNM community, but I have to be honest, the loneliness does not go away quickly. Finding a new social circle with like-minded people is more difficult than I would have thought, especially as we get further along in age. I know of a couple of people who are alcohol-free on my street, and I have reached out a little to them, but I think it may be time to start upping my game in the social arena. I'll never forget the quote from Johann Hari I used early in my blog:

"The opposite of addiction is not sobriety; the opposite of addiction is connection."

We need each other in this world of chaos and calamity. Something just hit me when I was typing the above quote, and this may not be true for everyone, but when I was drinking, I loved drinking alone. I would drink myself to sleep often, and I had no qualms about it. I am fairly certain I even passed on occasions to hang out with people because I preferred the idea of being alone and drinking. That breaks my heart a little.

Now that I am sober, I don't want to be alone as much. I miss the connection. I want to reach out and find people to converse and spend time with.

I am ready for human connection.

Are you?

Sober - Day 42

Thank God it's Alcohol-Free Friday, TGIAFF? Doesn't quite have the same ring to it, does it?

That is all right. You know what does have a nice ring to it? TGISAIANH—Thank God it's Saturday, and I am not hungover. Okay, maybe there is no ring to that at all, but at least there will not be ringing in my ears come tomorrow morning. I cannot even begin to express how much I do not miss the tired, foggy, headache-ridden mornings that followed nights of drinking. I also do not miss the middle of the night wake-ups, for who really knows what reason, I was experiencing to the point of sincere exhaustion during the months leading up to quitting. Sometimes, I feel like my head is so clear; it feels like my brain is spinning on overdrive, like it wants to accomplish all the things it was not allowed to accomplish during the decades of suppression I put it through. I want to keep up. I want to turn it loose and see what all I can conquer now that I can see clearly, again.

This, unfortunately, has begun to scare me a little.

The idea of overconfidence is beginning to tap me on the shoulder and ask me to acknowledge no matter how good everything feels or how confident I feel, life is a monster, and I cannot turn my back on her, ever. Think about it. Why did we start drinking in the first place? I am sure we all have a myriad of different reasons why, but I wonder if they stem from the same roots. In my first blog, I told you about my first experience drinking, but that was not why I began drinking. For me, I can look back and honestly say I was simply lost. My parents and family were known as the iconic perfect American family. Nevertheless, my parents split up my freshman year. My brothers were both gone, and my parents were busy re-establishing their own lives, so I think I felt abandoned on some level. I do not mean to use that as an excuse, but it is how I remember it. In fact, one of the things that has always bothered me is during that time, I have about a two-year period where I have very few memories. I have heard stories from both parents, teachers, and coaches I do not recall. What was I doing?

Whether it was drinking, smoking pot, or escaping through high school sports, surfing, or bicycle racing, I did whatever I could to hide from the reality that was clearly too much for me to handle alone. So, I found ways to hide. I found ways to not feel. I found ways to not deal with the things I did not want to deal with. Once the pattern started, it became easier and easier to lean on the thing that felt better than the other feelings I was feeling. And so, the behavior became established as the way I would deal with feelings of unease.

It all started with a feeling of unease, stress, unhappiness, loneliness, confusion, etc. Life, unfortunately, is filled with scenarios that can create any one of these feelings, as well as a number of others that could qualify in this category. So, if we allow ourselves to become overly confident in our way of life, isn't it possible we could let life get in the way as it did before? I don't know about you, but that is a terrifying thought and a thought I am not willing to allow to come to fruition.

The question, then, is how do we ensure we never allow ourselves to relax to the point of getting caught off-guard? How do we stay alert while continuing to reap the benefits of our new lives? How do we trust that no matter what life throws at us, we have learned enough to know better? How do we trust in ourselves and in our growth?

I think the answer just lies in our ability to see ourselves in a different way. So, essentially, the answer is once again perception. Our perception of ourselves is the key to our success. Am I now the kind of person that can have a curveball thrown at me and know how to adjust sufficiently to still hit it out of the park? A couple of months ago, I would have said no. But every day that goes by, and with each curve ball thrown my way, I am connecting and hitting the ball. Even if it is only a foul ball, I am still connecting. I am no longer swinging and hitting nothing but air. I have become a viable threat to the pitcher that is life.

SOBER - DAY 43

L and I got into a heated discussion regarding alcohol last night.

We just could not see the other's point of view, which was interesting because we were both bringing to the discussion similar enthusiasm, success, and ideas. We often engage in discussions since we quit about our experiences and mostly about how absurd it now feels to think we were ever in a difficult place with alcohol. At this point in time, it feels so far removed from our current reality. Nevertheless, we found ourselves in a violent, I say this lightly, disagreement about what alcohol is doing to society and why people begin drinking in the first place. After an agreed-upon reflection period from our discussion and combined with our newfound ability to engage in meaningful and fair conversation, we finally found what we believed to be the disconnect.

We were both approaching the discussion from opposite ends of the social spectrum. I think it took us a while to understand this because, at this point, we feel like equals, partners, and colleagues in this ever-changing match of life. But before we met, we came from very different backgrounds, and I am not even talking about upbringing, though that does have a slight role as well, I believe.

L was approaching the discussion from a place of "drinking to fit in." She did not grow up around alcohol-drinking parents or relatives. They drank some, but it was nothing of notice for her. She did not drink in high school, which is somewhat surprising considering the fitting-in piece. It was later, in adult life, where she started to feel the desire to want to be a part of a group. The people or group she was hoping to fit into consisted of professionals, self-proclaimed intellectuals, and "socialites." Her studies and career kept her moving and traveling so much she never really had the opportunity to create a close-knit friend group. So, when she had the opportunity to re-engage with her old friends and their friends who were, if you asked them, wine connoisseurs, it became the thing to do. They drank and talked about wine and all that went with the lifestyle, such as travel, food, events, and networking. She loved the fancy glasses, the environment, and the image that came with drinking wine. She was not drinking because she needed it; she was drinking because it was the thing to do and, of course, we all know what happens once we start drinking.

Her road to alcohol addiction was much different than mine.

In our conversation last night, it occurred to me my first experience with alcohol was not actually the infamous babysitting incident. It was even earlier. Earlier than twelve? For God's sake. Anyway, I was with my loose-cannon uncle in Portland, Oregon, during the Rose Festival. I don't fully remember the circumstances, but I do know beer (Schlitz) was involved and enough of it that I vaguely remember being sick. I do remember him laughing at me and my desperately hoping he thought I was cool. Thanks, Uncle. From there, I have a clear memory of why I began drinking. Even though I dabbled with it from time to time, it was more when my parents split up, and I felt I did not really belong anywhere that alcohol became one of my closest friends. I used it to make myself feel better. I used it to escape bad feelings. I used it not to be myself. This carried into adulthood. I did not drink to fit in, though I am sure I found people who drank, so my over-drinking did not stand out. Drinking for me was my way of self-medicating to feel better, pure and simple. Once it worked, it was my go-to any time I felt bad, sad, mad, lonely, depressed, happy, joyful, excited, celebratory. It helped me get through life, or so I thought.

Once we realized the disparity in the lenses we brought to the conversation, things began to make more sense, and we were able to have a more astute conversation about the differences in our experiences with alcohol. Another difference that came up, and one I might add was annoyingly accurate, was how we behaved differently while using alcohol. L, while drinking, still managed to be a very productive human. She said she often felt crappy and sometimes dropped the ball, but her version of dropping the ball was much different than mine. While she was checking off tasks on the weekends and getting things done, I often found it difficult to do anything at all. In fact, we often would argue about what we wanted our day to look like because L had an agenda, and I wanted no part of it. I just wanted to check out, as I called it, and so I did.

As I am writing this from yet another lens, the irony is astonishing. L is sitting next to me. I am writing a blog about my life experiences with alcohol; she is reading Quitlit, and I have Quitlit sitting next to me. We will both write, read, workout, probably clean the house, go snowboarding, make a healthy dinner, and more than likely make love. You know what's even better than that?

We will remember and enjoy every minute of it.

SOBER - DAY 44

Gratitude was the word of the day.

I took a beautiful picture on the drive up to Crystal Mountain this morning around 7:30 a.m. After taking the photograph, I couldn't help but think about all the reasons I feel so incredibly lucky to be alive and well.

The mountain was gorgeous today. While riding the lift on my way to the top of the mountain, I felt blessed for so many reasons. Just sitting there as I rose higher and higher up to the mountaintop, the sun was shimmering off the pure, white snow. The sky was cobalt blue, contrasting off the bright white of the mountain and peppered with emerald-green from the trees. The air was crisp and fresh, and the only sound you could really hear was the hum of the lift as the giant cable spun through the pulley system and the occasional scream of joy echoing off the mountain face. There was no way to feel anything other than joy and happiness.

I was sitting next to four other snow-loving people, but their experience seemed to be a little different. While I was reveling in the incredible natural beauty surrounding me, the other four people were pulling out flasks and bottles of Fireball whiskey. It was about 8:30 a.m., and these folks were already feeling the need to drown out something in the midst of all the surrounding beauty. The first thing that hit me was the fact they were me forty-five days ago. I remember last year heading up to Copper Mountain with a Colorado friend; we joked about hitting the bar first before heading up the first lift. We acted like we were joking, but I was not, and the only reason I didn't pursue it was I was not certain if our friend was joking or not either. Had she taken the reins, I would have followed her straight into the bar.

I do not want to sound like I am judging or putting down my lift mates; I just couldn't believe how strongly it hit me the seriousness of what is going on for people when they feel the need to drink so early and in the midst of so many beautiful and natural stimuli. I felt a little sad for them, and then I felt happy for myself because when they passed me the bottle, I simply said, "No thanks." That was it; I didn't offer my opinion or make any judgmental comments. I just declined, and ecstatically so. I wouldn't have traded what I was feeling for the world, let alone a drink I now know would quickly stifle the joy filling my soul.

I talked recently about how I have missed out on so many amazing life events because I was clouded in a haze of toxicity. Nothing gives me more pleasure than to think those days are over. I don't want to miss out on anything anymore. I don't even want to miss out on the crappy stuff, like in less than two weeks when I have to go back to court to defend myself from my ex. I want to be present because even the bad shit now has value to me. If I am fully present during the hard times, then I will truly appreciate the good times even more. I know this is a little cliche, but coming from a person who drowned out all the bad times, I did not have much to compare good times to when they did come, so it was anticlimactic.

Now I can see the difference, and the difference is magnificent.

In the vein of feeling grateful, I will finish with some of what I felt today up near the heavens. I am grateful for my son's health and wonderful temperament, for my wife and her never-ending support and love, for her health, for my son's health, for my health, for my job and the connections I build with students, for my beautiful home and badass car, for my incredibly patient and understanding therapist, for my courage to take on this new path, for my dedication to writing, for my love of photography, for my friends and family, and for my new life.

I am grateful.

Sober - Day 45

If human connection really is the opposite of addiction, as Johan Hari states, then isn't it important to define human connection?

The dictionary defines connection, in its simplest form, as something that connects. It also references a contextual relation or association, a causal or logical relation, and, of course, intimate, social, and professional relationships. With this in mind, though, almost every aspect of our lives deals with a human connection. Which human connections are we in need of to support a healthier, more fulfilled life, especially when quitting an addiction?

Interestingly, I believe if you asked one hundred people what kind of connection they are lacking in their lives preventing them from feeling fulfilled, you would receive a myriad of different answers. This, I believe, is due to the fact humans possess a diverse array of wants and needs, and they are all interdependent upon the individual's personal character, background, personality, friendships, knowledge, and even socioeconomic background. Depending on the person, the human connection desired may be vastly different.

How do we define our individual needs for human connection?

I think this is an incredibly poignant question, and one I have not heard spoken about at great length since I have embarked on the alcohol-free lifestyle. This is most likely due to what I stated in the previous paragraph—there is no one answer that fits all. It's individual, personal, intimate, and probably a little scary for us to admit what we need. But, we have to, don't we?

Over the past couple of years, I think I have known this was an issue for me. It was not because I do not have an amazing partner. I am not miserable at my job. I am not unhappy as a parent. I just never really learned how to be alone, how to thrive by myself, or how to be happy in my own skin. I know I have tried to reach out and create connections, not always successfully, but I have tried. Now that my mind is clearer, and I am trying to allow myself to be more aware, I am beginning to see the problem in the past was I did not know what connections I wanted to create. I kept trying to force connections that, maybe, were not the most beneficial to either party. This is not to say I did not appreciate every person who has crossed paths with me; I think we learn from every connection. I am saying I believe I am ready to begin creating stronger connections, and more importantly, I am ready to be a stronger connection for others, too.

What am I hoping to find? I think it is actually pretty simple. I would like to find a couple of people—it would be great if they were couples so L and I both could benefit—who share our passions, who are intellectual, who enjoy conversation, who are sober, who like to stay in touch, and who like to spend time with positive people, not complain about how busy or hard life is. I want to surround myself with some people who push me to be better, stronger, and better as a friend.

This sounds like a dating profile, but all I am really saying is I am ready to build some strong, productive, equitable, and fulfilling relationships.

I am ready for human connection built from a foundation of growth and acceptance.

Sober - Day 46

Systemic peer pressure.

I have read a lot lately from people posting on the TNM community page about how someone has passed on attending an event, hanging out with friends, or traveling because they do not want to deal with having to tell people they are not drinking.

This is a horrific burden.

Think about the absurdity of this belief. I—a person who is allowing myself to become more aware, who is trying to better myself, make my body and mind more healthy, who is trying to think outside the norm, make better decisions, improve the life of my family, be a better role model for my kids, be a better friend, spouse, parent, employee, colleague—am afraid to do something I enjoy because there will be people present who may make fun of me, not understand me, or will at least force me to feel like I have to justify why I am not drinking poison. In what other context on this planet does this kind of systemic peer pressure occur to an evolved, highly intelligent, free-thinking, educated population? It doesn't, ever.

I know I have felt the concern about how to deal with outings around people who are drinking, but I have had a much better time dealing with this than a lot of people I have been following. For me, I was so fed up with my drinking I simply did not care what somewhat else thought about my unwillingness to partake in libations. The first time I did it and realized nobody really cared, I then spent the rest of the evening enjoying the social experiment that is inhabiting a group of drinkers as the sole sober person. I found I actually enjoyed the scenario more than I would have thought. It was fascinating to me, and I experienced no fear of missing out, as they say, and on the contrary, felt like I was the only one who wasn't.

I understand the concern, though. It can feel weird, especially when you take into account the somber "sorries" and pouting lips as people try to act the way they are "supposed" to act around someone who is making a life choice that is positively benefiting the rest of their lives and the lives of everyone around them.

Why do people feel the need to feel bad for us?

I guess it is part of the systemic problem. We have been taught if someone can't handle alcohol, *they* have a problem. It can't be that everyone has the ability to become addicted to one of the most highly addictive substances on the planet, and it really isn't anyone's fault. In fact, it is probably more accurate to say those making pouty faces and apologizing are really the ones who are having the hardest time. I know when I was drinking way too much, I found ways to justify my drinking, and one of the ways I did that was by finding people to hang out with who drank so I didn't have to feel bad about the amount I drank. That's what we do; it is part of the systemic problem.

We make each other feel better for our behaviors. We distance ourselves from people who seem to "have it together" because that would be too close to home; don't we all want to figure out how to live a better, more fulfilling life? Of course, we do, but when we are drowning in our own frustration for not being able to, we do not want to be reminded it is possible. It reminds me of a quote from a cheesy eighties movie, *Days of Thunder*, when the crew chief tells Tom Cruise's girlfriend, "You will never see a race car driver at a funeral until he is actually dead; it reminds him of what can happen." I think this is true for us when we are stuck in a cycle of drinking. We want to get better, but when we believe we can't, we avoid anything suggesting otherwise. It makes it easier.

What is the answer to alcoholic systemic peer pressure?

We need to all be there for each other. TNM community is really good at this. It allows people to vent frustrations and cheer accomplishments. People seem to honestly care about those who take the step to reach out. They offer advice, experience, and a shoulder if needed. We need more of this, but we need it in our real world, too.

It's difficult to find sober people these days, probably because we are all too afraid to tell anyone we do not drink.

I do not drink alcohol. Want to hang out?

SOBER - DAY 47

It is *all* about lifestyle choices.

The last big piece of the puzzle for me on this journey is retraining my mind to see working out as a lifestyle, not something I have to do. I get started with a couple of days in a row and start to feel pretty good about myself, then something comes up and distracts me for a week, and I lose my momentum and have to start all over again. The starting all over again is excruciating for me, to be honest. I just need to find a way to make it a priority. I have done it before with diet; why can't I do it with exercise?

About twenty years ago, I made a pretty rash decision to give up eating meat. There were several reasons, but mostly it was because I was deep into scuba diving at the time, and I had fallen in love with sea creatures of all varieties. I still remember the day it hit me. I was diving off the coast of

Monterey Bay in California. I came upon a ledge on the ocean floor that held a small cavern behind it. On the ledge, there were several shrimp lined up on the ledge, and this caught my attention. As I swam up to the ledge to get a closer look, I noticed the shrimp lined up on the ledge started moving around spastically. As I got even closer, the shrimps started doing flips, over and over; they were jumping up and down and running from side to side. I remember laughing through my regulator at that bizarre sight. After a few moments of watching the underwater circus, I noticed something else, and this simple visual changed my life for the past twenty years. Behind the flipping, seemingly crazy shrimp were a bunch of babies. They were all huddled up together in a loose ball. The adult shrimp were trying to protect them. I am six feet, three inches tall and weigh over 180 pounds, and these tiny creatures took it upon themselves to protect their young at all costs. Why was this so meaningful to me? Because we think of sea creatures as having no feelings, we have been told they have no nerves, so they can't feel, but there in front of me were a bunch of adult shrimp protecting their babies. They feel something.

At that point, I gave up eating seafood, and shortly thereafter, I decided, *why eat meat at all*, so I gave up eating the rest of the flesh in the world, too. It was personal; it mattered enough to me to make a massive lifestyle change, and I have never looked back. By the way, I am not one to preach my dietary beliefs to others. I even cooked Thanksgiving day turkey for the family a couple of years in a row. It is simply my belief, and I live the lifestyle for me.

So, now I am trying to incorporate the same way of thinking toward working out. I am an active person anyway, snowboarding, walking, biking, etc., but I have struggled to make it a priority on a daily basis. The interesting part of this to me is, now that I am sober, getting up and working out in the morning should be even easier. I don't feel like crap, and I have more energy. Nevertheless, it has still been a little difficult for me to commit to. I know I'll get there; with all I have conquered in the past couple of months, there is no doubt but I can be a little impatient.

Last year, L and I rode the Seattle to Portland (STP) bike ride in two days. It was two hundred miles, one hundred miles per day. I had barely trained but did it anyway. We had a great time, but it was difficult. This year, I made a goal to ride the STP in one day—two hundred miles in one day. L is going to do it with me as well. I am bringing this up to proclaim my goal to anyone willing to listen in the hopes of encouraging myself to keep my training going. It has been a little hit-and-miss since January, but this morning, I got up early and rode for the third day in a row, which is progress.

I know this has not been as much about alcohol as my other posts, but in a way, it is all about alcohol. The reason I did not train last year for the two-day STP was because I was hungover all the time and could never get the motivation to workout. This year, not only am I already training more, but I also made a decision to make it even harder on myself, doing it in one day, because I know I am in a better mental place to physically prepare for the big day. Also, quitting alcohol is probably going to make the one-day, two-hundred-mile bike ride easier than the two-day ride last year because my body will not be working from a constant state of dehydration and exhaustion. I guess we will see.

The bottom line for me is this: In order to make any meaningful change, it will most likely have to come from a place of perception. We have to change the way we think about ourselves and the thing we are hoping to change.

SOBER - DAY 48

Setting and achieving goals.

I can't remember if I mentioned this in this blog yet, but I set a pretty lofty goal for myself about a month ago. One of the things I gave up during the last six or so years of my drinking days was writing. That is why this blog became so important to me. One of the goals I set the day I quit drinking was to blog about it every day for thirty days. After those thirty days ended, I did not want to quit writing about it, so here I am, still blogging about my experience every day for forty-eight days.

Another goal I set once I started writing again was to finally start writing another novel. I started feeling so good about my dedication to my blog, I began to believe it was time to embark on another novel-writing journey. I have written two other books, the first in my early thirties and before I even made the decision to go to college, and the second after I began my literature studies at the University of Washington. I am proud of both, even if they were not ready to see or be accepted by the harsh and critical publishing world out there. Nevertheless, how many people can say they have written two novels? I have!

Once I began writing my third novel, I decided I needed to make a deadline for myself. The book aligns with my reluctant desire to remove myself from therapy as well. I figured if I stay on the path I am currently on until my birthday, April 30, I will feel confident enough that I have the tools necessary to pursue my sober and nicotine-free life on my own. So, to add weight to my decision, I decided to make the goal to finish my first draft of the novel I am writing for my birthday as well. If all goes as planned, I will be out of therapy with a completed novel and still alcohol and nicotine-free. Woohoo! I cannot lie and say this does not scare me because it does. I have been seeing my therapist for over a year now, and she has been one of the most influential people I have ever had in my life. But, at some point, I need to leave the nest and go out on my own. Thankfully, I have an amazing support system at home too, but it will be another step in my growth and emotional discipline. I'll be ready.

Laura McKowen, author of *We Are the Luckiest*, sends out emails if you want them about random ideas and experiences she has. Today, I received one from her that talked about "tying the dog to the fucking tree." What I loved about this was first, how timely it is for me, but also how we can relate the idea of the dog to any aspect of our lives keeping us from accomplishing the things we want to accomplish. For me, the dog I need to tie to the tree is my desire to make everything happen yesterday. Even as I began writing my novel, I couldn't help but think about how to get people interested in my book and what steps I needed to take in case it's good enough to try and publish. My dog is my need to chill the fuck out, enjoy the process, have fun with the writing, be patient, and wait until it is time to take the next steps. The next steps will arrive and present themselves when they are ready. Today, I am tying my "dog" to a tree.

What is your "dog"?

Sober - Day 49

What is agency and is it relevant to recovery?

This term came up over dinner last night with L. We were talking about what we are reading, both from our Quitlit and our novels. She mentioned the word agency, and this immediately dredged up memories of my literature studies at the University of Washington. Agency was a buzzword at the time, and to be honest, I became tired of hearing about it. Last night, however, the word created different feelings for me, now that I have dealt with more of life's struggles and discovered more reasons and needs to stand up for myself or take care of my family. Then, I thought about how it relates to alcohol or any addiction.

First, let's take a look at the meaning of the word, agency:

a. The office or function of an agent.
b. The relationship between a principal and that person's agent.

c. The capacity, condition, or state of acting or of exerting power.

d. A person or thing through which power is exerted or an end is achieved. (Dictionary.com)

The first two definitions do not do much for me, but they are relevant to how we can use agency in our lives. An agent can be a person who works for an individual to achieve or gain a certain goal or thing. The agent, in this case, does whatever is reasonably necessary to obtain the desired goal. The person whom the agent works for simply pays them and sits back and waits for the goal to come to fruition.

I don't know about any of you, but I have never been in a position to hire an agent to do anything for me, and especially not to help quit drinking.

Let's look at definition three (c): the capacity, condition, or state of acting or of exerting power. Now we are talking about some higher-level thinking. The capacity, meaning the ability to do something; the condition and state, meaning from a position; to exert power, meaning to do something for ourselves that may be bigger than how we perceive ourselves to be (there is that damn word again). In this context, agency comes from within. How are we paying this agent? We are paying with our pride, fear, anxiety, embarrassment, shame, self-loathing, or simply our need for change. By acknowledging any or all of these emotions and feelings, we are giving ourselves the ability to emotionally afford the agent living within us and telling them to go out and fight for what we are seeking.

Agency in recovery is paramount to success. We have to know we have the ability to change. We have to know we have the strength. We have to know we are our own best advocates, promoters, and agents for getting us exactly whatever it is we need or want. In this case, sobriety, but what else can our agency do for us? What can our agency do for those around us? What can our agency do for our society? I believe it is endless, but it all begins with . . . wait for it . . . our perception of what we believe we are capable of. We all have an agent living deep within us, just waiting, begging, pleading to come out. We just have to let them.

I invited my agent to come out recently, and she is a badass!

Sober - Day 50

"Lost time is never found again." (Benjamin Franklin)

I got up this morning, on a Saturday, at 6:00 a.m., and rallied up the family for a trip to Crystal Mountain for a day of snowboarding. I had a rough couple of days with ex drama, and I have court this coming Thursday, so I needed a good day on the mountain to unwind. The family woke up like champs, and we headed up to the hill for yet another one of our crazy adventures. The conditions were pretty good, and we had a lot of fun tearing up the mountain as a family. It's actually pretty awesome to see us shredding down the hillside with thirty-eight years separating us and each one of us having just as much fun as the other. I always feel a little blessed when I am carving up the snow or taking jumps, and I see L and X next to me, ahead of me, or behind me. I love sharing the space with them.

While on the mountain, the subject of time came up. For me, the mention of this word is visceral. I literally feel a chill overtake my senses when I hear it now that I am sober. I think it is probably a little bit like kryptonite for anyone in recovery. For each of us, it may be different, but on some level, I am willing to bet we all can relate to some common conceptions about time.

What did time mean to me then?

Time has not been my best friend. I can say with certainty time was a big part of my downfall with each and every one of my addictions. You see, time meant having to face all the feelings I was able to avoid while working, sleeping, keeping active, or other activities that distracted me. But those distractions were only that, distractions. They distracted my thoughts from the real emotions and feelings that came from living and simply being human. I cannot avoid the reality life will create stress, pain, heartache, loss, anxiety, uncertainty, and any other of a thousand things I will face on a daily basis. When I am busy, I do not have to think about any of those things. But when I am still, when I have time on my hands, my mind naturally wants to redirect toward those life issues because it knows if I do not deal with them soon, they will build up and overtake my ability to deal with anything else in my daily life.

Unless . . .

I drown those feelings with chemicals: nicotine, alcohol, drugs, sex, food, etc. Any of these addictive substances put all of those unwanted feelings and emotions on hold indefinitely. As long as I was using, my internal need to heal was suspended. Unfortunately, while on this holding pattern for emotional growth and healing, I also lost an immense amount of time off my life. I don't even mean in terms of health, which is also true. I mean in terms of just minutes, hours, days, weeks, months, and years where I probably did a lot of really cool activities and saw a lot of really incredible scenery, shows, and performances. I probably met some amazing people and had quality time with my family and friends. I potentially lost all of those experiences forever so I could indulge my ridiculous need to suppress my true feelings and emotions. I can never get that time back.

What does time mean to me now?

It means everything. I have never spent such quality time with myself, with my family, in my job, with my friends, with my hobbies, and with my dreams. I have more time now than I have ever had because I am not choosing to drown time with something that does nothing but take time away from me. I have evenings where I have done so much throughout the day and night that I can't believe I still have time left before bed, and then I have to think of how I want to spend that time, too. That is a dilemma I have never experienced in my entire life, but that is a dilemma I am learning to love and cherish each and every time I experience it. Give me more time; I now know how to spend it wisely.

If someone asked me, "What is the single greatest benefit you have found from giving up alcohol?" I would say with certainty, "Time!"

Sober - Day 51

"Letting go of exhaustion as a status symbol." (Brené Brown)

Sitting on the sofa during a sober Sunday morning writing in my novel, L read me the above quote. Damn! It hit me like a two-by-four across the face. I haven't read the book she was quoting, but I may after hearing that quote; it's called *The Gifts of Imperfection*. I don't even know what Brene has to say about it yet. I just stopped everything I was doing and said, "I need to write about that."

I see things so incredibly different since giving up alcohol. If I'm completely honest, it is actually quite annoying. Ignorance is bliss is not so far off the mark. Before I gave up drinking, I didn't have to acknowledge all the crazy happening around me on a daily basis. I was able to just check out and pretend it all did not apply to me. I was able to ignore all the absurdities I saw around me and live in my bubble of alcohol-induced apathy. Of course, I am joking about it being annoying, but awareness can be somewhat taxing.

Why did the above quote hit me so hard?

You hear it every day and everywhere you go. You hear it at your job, at home, at the grocery store, on television, in the movies, in books, everywhere. Somewhere along the line, we decided being overly busy is important to who we are as a person. If you are not busy, you must not be very important. It is a keeping up with the Joneses mentality, isn't it?

I remember when I went to college full time at the age of thirty-seven. I was married, working full-time as a bartender, and had a baby. I don't remember ever feeling busier than I did at that moment in my life. I mean, seriously. I had not one moment of extra time; granted, it was by choice. Nevertheless, I also don't remember ever being more irritated with the eighteen to twenty-two-year-olds who would proclaim how busy and exhausting their lives were during class or in the library during study time. My jaw would hit the table, and I would chuckle to myself and think, *oh my, do you have an eye-opening experience coming your way in the very near future.* I don't think I meant it in a judgmental way, but more in a are-you-fucking-kidding-me kind of way.

The point being, even at the age of eighteen, these kids are learning they are expected to act like they do so much they just can't take on one more thing. Where and why did this become such a thing?

I wonder if it relates to alcohol. You can roll your eyes at that one if you wish but think about it. What does alcohol do to all of us? It lowers our drive, makes us lazy, forces us to trudge through our days after nights of drinking. It lowers our expectations, makes us disregard things that might normally bother us, keeps us in a haze of toxic uniformity. The more we allow ourselves to live in this state, the less we are capable of accomplishing, so what better way to excuse our lack of motivation and drive? Proclaim how much we are doing so nobody is ever aware of how little we are actually achieving.

I am aware this is a slight generalization, but honestly, tell me that there is not some truth to this. I know, now that I am sober and changing the way I see my life and the world around me, I do not feel exhausted. I am taking on new things every day. I am excited I have more to give and I want to achieve all my goals. I do not need to tell anyone how tired I am; on the contrary, I have been writing for fifty-one days about how fucking good I feel, and after decades of feeling the opposite,

I am not going to let anyone take that away from me. And nor should you.

Let's make "I feel amazing!" the new normal.

Sober - Day 52

This is going to be a difficult week.

I have to go back to court on Thursday regarding things that still need to be resolved with my ex. I am not trying to dump my shit on anyone who has taken the time to read this, but I am attempting to let anyone who is reading this know I do have a tough week coming up, and I am human. I am taking the day off work Thursday to attend the hearing. Regardless of how it goes, it should be the end of it for a while. I am putting open and positive energy out to whoever is involved with this case.

I struggle with waiting around to see what is going to happen next. L is struggling with it too, and we keep telling ourselves there is nothing more we can do, but as I said, we are human, and we struggle just like everyone else when life throws difficult situations our way. All I know for certain is I could do little else to be a great father to my son. He loves me, he loves L, and we have a great little family. One day, I just hope he ends up with me full-time.

In the meantime, I am going to continue doing what I do. Writing, working, spending quality time with L and X, and working toward a wonderful, sober, and fulfilling life. Come Thursday, I will just show up and take what is given me and then move the fuck on. Finally!

In the spirit of sticking to my goals and the positive and honest lifestyle I am living, I slipped on one of my goals this weekend, and I am trying not to beat myself up over it. Writing has been what I believe to be the catalyst for everything positive happening in my life right now. I wrote last week about goals, and one of the goals I made was to write in my novel every day so I have a rough draft by my birthday on April 30. This weekend, with snowboarding and X's visit, I did not write over the weekend. So, now I am two days behind, which means I have three days' worth of writing to do to get caught up. It may not seem like a big deal, but it is to me because I have been trying to stay dedicated to my goals. I have kept the blog going because, for some reason, I feel it is important to me and my sober journey. I hope someone out there is still enjoying it.

I had a thought about my blog this weekend, though. I think I am going to keep it going for one hundred days straight and then compile them all into a book and see what happens. I figure, why not. It has been incredibly healing for me; maybe others will feel the same way. I like the thought, but more importantly, I like that it keeps me motivated to write every day.

Who knows what can happen and, like Russell Wilson says, why not [me]?

Sober - Day 53

It's okay to have a bad day too, right?

I've talked a little bit about this before, but one of the most interesting aspects of living a sober life for me is how my perception has changed on what I see as acceptable behavior or not. I am on day fifty-three, which is an amazing accomplishment considering how much I had been drinking and how much I told myself I didn't really have a problem. But, at the same time, I am really just a baby in the sober world. I forget this because, in just fifty-three days, my whole world has changed for the better.

A year and a few months ago, I began therapy to make some changes. I wanted to work on three things I considered addictions, but I did not really have a plan for what that looked like. I wanted to replace those addictions with things I stopped doing that made me happy and, on a simpler note, I just wanted to be a better man.

In the past fifty-three days, I have essentially quit, not just worked on, three addictions, and I have begun incorporating again all of the healthy things that bring joy into my life. I am writing every day, doing photography, working out every day, and pursuing a life beyond what I currently know and have accepted. When I talked with my therapist last night, I began crying when I talked about how far I have come in such a short period of time. It's emotional because it has been life-changing and such a positive experience for me. The only thing left to do is keep on track and then add in all the aspects of life I never thought I was worthy of because now I know I am worthy.

This morning, I woke up feeling heavy. Granted, I have some stuff going on this week that is dragging me down a little, and rightly so. But, with all the positive that is happening, I sometimes forget that I am still merely human, and I am going to have bad days. I am going to experience things that don't feel good, that piss me off, that make me sad, that make me want to throw something. I know all this, but since I quit drinking and have experienced this new side of me, I feel a little indestructible. I feel like I should not experience those feelings anymore. As unrealistic as that is, I don't even know if it bothers me I feel this way. I have spent a lifetime feeling like nobody, like someone who deserves all the bad things that come my way, and like a less important version of myself.

When these days happen, and I'm feeling low or heavy, is it okay not to accept them? What do highly positive and successful people do with these days? This is all new to me. In the past, I didn't even acknowledge them as bad days; they were just normal for me, and the way I dealt with them was, well, you know. Now, I notice them. I notice the hell out of them, and I do not like them. It makes me want to throw down with those feelings and say, "You are not welcomed here anymore."

But I know that is not the best way to handle them.

So, I am just doing what I do with any of the twinges of feelings that come up regarding any of my past beliefs. I sit with them. I acknowledge them as a memory from a past version of myself. I recognize them as something I no longer desire to have in my life. Then, I move on.

This blog is me moving on.

Thanks for letting me vent a little. Today is going to be another amazingly positive, productive, happy, and sober day.

Here's to a new perspective on bad days.

Sober - Day 54

What is the most beneficial aspect of living alcohol-free?

I have seen a lot of posts, tweets, and talk about why living alcohol-free is so amazing. I think it is interesting how, for most of us who read TNM, there was a new take on the idea of quitting alcohol. It came from a new perspective, which helped a lot of us see giving up alcohol as a reward and not a punishment. For me, it was honestly as easy as making a decision to use olive oil over canola oil. Once I learned one was better for me than the other, I just said, "okay," and made the change. Thinking about alcohol as a poison really made the connection, for me, to how ignorant drinking is for our body and mind.

Unfortunately, not everyone is making the same connection.

As I read through everyone's posts, blogs, and tweets every day, I realize how differently we all respond to the idea of giving up alcohol. I honestly can't believe I went from drinking as much as I did to nothing, nada, nil, overnight. I just didn't want it anymore. L and I have talked about how, for us, it might have just been the exact right moment, and thankfully, we listened to that urging inside our body and mind. But I still remember the immense conflict floating around inside my brain for years, knowing I was drinking too much but not wanting to either admit it or give it any credibility. Getting to where I am today did not happen overnight, even though it feels that way once I made the decision. I went through countless attempts at quitting. I fought with partners, beat myself up for driving when I should not have, I regretted missing out on events I was not-so-present for, I said things I shouldn't have, I did things I shouldn't have, I went to work feeling like death, I have started unnecessary confrontations because I wasn't thinking clearly, and I have argued countless times how I did not have a problem with alcohol.

This was not an easy road, until it was.

What is the best aspect of living alcohol-free? Where do I start? There are a myriad of reasons I could state to support giving up alcohol, but I am only going to concentrate on the three I think are the most important, from my experience.

Confidence. I have walked through my life for forty-eight years living with low self-esteem, unsure of who I was or what I was meant to do, afraid of making mistakes, embarrassed about my ideas, and certain I did not deserve positive outcomes in my life. People who know me may not be aware of all this, but that is the beauty of internal conflict. It's internal, and we can go our entire lives fighting a battle nobody even knows is occurring. I was good at hiding my battles from the outside world. When you become aware people use alcohol to hide from their internal battles, then it becomes painfully obvious battles are raging all around us every day. What I have gained in confidence from giving up alcohol is almost too much to articulate in words. I do not feel like the same man I was only two months ago. I see the world differently now. I expect good things to happen to me, and when they don't, I can deal with them better. I know what I am worth, and let me tell you, we are all worth so much more than we ever knew while using. I am pursuing passions I gave up due to low self-esteem, and I love them more than I ever did before

I quit. Confidence in and of itself is a wonderful thing to gain back. I had no idea how much I was missing out.

Time. This one caught me off guard; I was not expecting to gain as much time as I have gained over the past fifty-four days. I figured, yeah, I spent time drinking in the evenings and weekends, etc., but was I really wasting all that much time? As it turns out, I was wasting all of my time, and it was because of my drinking. It was not just the actual action of pouring drinks down my throat that wasted so much time. It was the time after I began drinking that really mattered. As soon as I took my first drink, I lost my motivation to do pretty much anything except drink more. So then the course was set for the rest of the evening or day if I began early. I would find things to do that supported drinking and nothing that didn't, like working out, reading, writing, photography, or any number of things I stopped doing once my drinking amped up. It was not only the day I drank where I lost time, but it was also the next day when I was hungover and unmotivated to do anything that day either. This would last until the evening, when I finally had the opportunity to have another drink to mask the pain caused by the previous day. It was a horrific cycle of self-deprivation. Once I started living alcohol-free, I gained all that time back. I have engaged in all my passions with a fervor of which I never knew I was capable. I am completing every goal I set, I am creating new goals every day, and I am living a life full of time. How amazing is it to go through the day with energy, excitement, and a positive attitude about your future? To me, it is everything.

Connection. This beneficial aspect has so many layers. Going back to Johann Hari's coined phrase, "The opposite of addiction is not sobriety; the opposite of addiction is connection," I believe this is one of the most amazing things a person can gain from living a sober life. While connection in Johann Hari's speech was geared more toward human connection, I think connection can mean so many things. Connection to a belief, to words, to hobbies, to beauty, to yourself, to life, or simply to freedom can be as beneficial as any human connection. I do not intend to diminish human connection because obviously, it is incredibly important too, but I believe when we begin to smother our real selves with chemicals, food, work, sex, or anything else that masks reality, we lose connection with things we love as well as people. Those things can make the difference between being happy and feeling worthless. When I went to therapy a little over a year ago, my therapist asked me what I saw myself doing if I was not engaging in addictive behaviors. My answer: reading, writing, photography, exercise, family, friends, and feeling better about myself.

What have I achieved over the past fifty-four days? All of the above.

Sober - Day 55

I cannot change the outcome of today's events.

I woke up at 4:30 a.m., unable to sleep. I have been pretty stressed out this past week, thinking of all the things that have occurred to bring me to this point. Questions pile up in my head: What did I do wrong? What could I have done differently? How is this going to turn out? What does it mean about me if it does not go my way? Will I be able to handle a loss? When those questions started to come to a head, I felt anxiety take over and pull me down. It makes me feel powerless and helpless. The problem at this point is I have done everything I can do, and now, it is simply up to the judge hearing the case to decide what is right, just, and fair.

L got up with me and will be attending the hearing as well for moral support. She is just as invested at this point as I am. X and her are close and have been from day one. I put on a tie and looked at myself in the mirror, and it occurred to me I am okay this morning. Here we are, on the day of the hearing, and I feel good. I am sober, clear-headed, looking sharp, and feeling positive. No matter how this thing turns out, I will be fine, and X and I will continue to maintain our amazing relationship, even from a thousand miles away. Life is good.

I have been talking with two new sober friends for the past week or so via text. We met through our sober journeys. I am amazed at how things are working out for all of us. They, too, have been struggling with life issues outside of sobriety. A common thread I keep seeing with them and everyone else I have come into contact with since I quit drinking is that things tend to work out. I don't know if it is the perception we hold is different regarding situations or if our perceptions are changing the outcomes of the situations, but whatever it is, it seems life leans in favor of those who are living well.

Now, I am not totally naive. I know today may not go my way, but I also know no matter what happens, I will be able to handle the outcome. I know this because I am feeling stronger than I have ever felt, I am making better life choices, I am allowing positivity to exist in my heart, and I am more open to love than ever before. Once this is over, the outcome will not change or negatively affect any of these qualities in my life.

I am going to keep this a little shorter today, as I am needing to head out the door to my hearing. I hope everyone is flooded with love, peace, and acceptance today. I am always here for anyone who is on this journey; please allow yourself to be there for others as well.

Live light.

Sober - Day 56

Yet, another new chapter.

In an attempt to not bore you with details, I will say this. Yesterday could have gone better, but it could have gone much, much worse. The court landed us somewhere in the middle of all the chaos being deliberated. Which, in all honesty, is about as fair an outcome as I could have realistically hoped. I am at least able to walk away from it feeling as though I was heard and not completely taken advantage of. The judge, at one point, actually said, "The amount of travel you do and the amount of time you spend with your son is incredible; kudos to you, Dad."

I couldn't agree more.

So, with that year-and-a-half battle wrapped up and tied with a nice little bow on it, I am happy to move forward, knowing I can let go of most of the negativity associated with that awful situation and just concentrate on being a dad and enjoying my son. Speaking of which, I am jumping on a plane this afternoon to go to California to pick him up and then head to Big Bear Mountain for some snowboarding tomorrow. I am hoping for a very uncrowded mountain since, well, you know [this was in regard to the beginning of the pandemic]. I was going to go boarding after the hearing yesterday, but it ran too long, and we didn't get a chance to make it up to Crystal Mountain. Boarding tomorrow is a very much needed activity for me, and I can't wait to get up there and enjoy some snow and nature.

When I got home yesterday, I received an email from my school district stating they are canceling all schools for six weeks. I have no idea what this means, but I am pretty sure it does not mean I will not work for six weeks. I do think I will have some spare time on my hands. This, in conjunction with all I have been working toward since becoming sober, will be nice timing. I plan to use the extra time to dig deeper into my writing and be as productive as I possibly can. Mostly, it virtually assures me of making my April 30 deadline of completing the rough draft for my novel. After putting writing off for over six years, it is somewhat unfathomable to comprehend I will have written a book in less than three months, and even more so considering it is all because of a much-needed decision to quit drinking. Sober life is fucking amazing.

Along with the writing vein of this blog, I have some other potentially exciting news. I have been asked to edit a memoir for a friend. It is a paid gig, and it will be helpful for me in my writing as well as in preparing me for the publishing journey I have coming my way when I finish my two books. I am constantly amazed by how the positive energy I am feeling and exerting is coming back to me with every step I take down this new path of my life. What is even more amazing is I actually feel and believe I deserve it, and I have never in my life been able to say that.

I have a cousin who made a comment to me once when I asked what she attributed to the positive events occurring in her life. She simply said, "Living well." Is it really that simple? Is that how we bring positivity, good luck, and good fortune into our lives? We just live well? Where the fuck was I when this memo was handed out? The memo I received was more like, just do the best you can with whatever you're given, and don't be afraid to drown yourself in your misery because life is really fucking hard.

Well, it may be a day late and a dollar short, but I finally got the first memo, and I am graciously accepting and enacting the challenge to simply live well.

Want to join me?

Sober - Day 57

I flew down to California to pick up my son last night, and then we drove out to San Bernardino to stay the night before heading up to Big Bear Mountain this morning. I won't lie and say I did not drive around for a little while looking for a place that sold non-alcoholic beer. I mean, it was Friday night. I didn't have any luck, so we checked into the hotel and went to bed early.

I woke up this morning too early. My head was still spinning from the court decision, and even though I am doing my best to be positive, it is difficult to hear someone lie about you.

Anyway.

I woke up early and decided to write a little before heading up to the mountain. I am sitting here at 6 a.m. on a Saturday morning, feeling as clear-headed and awake as I could possibly feel. Now that I have been sober for going on two months, I am already taking for granted, slightly, the unbelievable gift of waking up in the morning and *never* feeling miserable or disgusted with myself. I cannot wait to get on the mountain and snowboard with my son on what looks to be a very good day for snowboarding in California.

I was contacted by a newly sober friend when I landed yesterday. We met sobriety, and we have been chatting via text for a couple of weeks now. She was having a little trouble yesterday with her desire to drink. She said it just sounded good, which we all can relate to, and it is hard to argue the feeling when you are still in that unstable place with alcohol. I tried to remind her of a couple of things that have really flipped the switch for me in the whole idea of missing alcohol.

First, the single biggest idea that stuck with me after reading TNM was when Annie said alcohol is the only drug we have to make an excuse not to do. Once I heard that statement , I could not unhear it. The stigma associated with drinking, and especially with the idea that some people "have a problem," actually started to piss me off. There should never be a situation, from a social standpoint, where someone has to feel bad about trying to live healthier. That is a taught and learned behavior orchestrated over the last two centuries of alcohol-related history. I will never feel bad or make an excuse for not wanting to poison myself.

Secondly, people who are still drinking began to pique my interest. One of the things that started to really reach down deep inside me was when I started watching, and more importantly, listening to those who are still drinking. Let me be clear. I do not think I am better than anyone because I don't drink. I am simply more aware of some things than I used to be while drinking Once I started watching people drink, I mean, really watching, I started to realize all the things I have done in my past and how stupid I must have made myself look over the years while drinking alcohol. The things people say and the slurring manner in which they say them is shocking to witness. Unwarranted confidence begins to creep into dialogue. Unnecessary arguments begin to unfold throughout the night. There is an inability for people to listen to another's point of view because they are barely hanging on to their own. While witnessing all of these things take place, it is hard to ignore the fact alcohol degrades our intellect and ability to cope with normal social situations.

Lastly, I cannot say enough about how wonderful it is to *never* wake up feeling like crap. To *never* wake up wondering if you said something you might regret. To *never* wonder if you did something you may have to pay for. To *never* struggle to remember what happened over the course of an evening. There is so much joy in beginning a day feeling confident, positive, healthy, and happy. With that said, I wish to impart the following very simple statement, one that should be trending in the world this morning, to my newly sober friends:

Happy Sober Saturday! Go get some productive shit done.

SOBER - DAY 58

Let's show kindness and build connections.

I am stuck in a hotel room. Stuck is not the right word, but you know what I mean. I am with my ten-year-old son and we are trying to find ways to entertain ourselves during these crazy times. I have to drop him off at 2:00 p.m. and then catch another empty plane home. I have heard there is a consideration of canceling domestic travel, which is heartbreaking for me because that means I may not be able to visit my son for an extended period of time. I made a promise to him, over four years ago, I would never go longer than two weeks between visits (and that only after two consecutive weekly visits), but now it seems I may be made a liar. I know he will understand, but it does not make it any easier for either of us.

While he is doing his thirty-minute reading time, I am writing my daily blog about my experiences with sobriety.

Unrelated thought: if everyone started reading again, due to the potential shutdown, books could make a resurgence, which would be perfect timing considering I will be completing two books by the end of April.

Anyway, I have been thinking a lot about how kindness has seemingly taken a back seat to personal agendas these days. When I try to impart what little wisdom I have to my son, it generally revolves around kindness and awareness. I think if we can hold on to even just those two ideals, we could change the world. I know there are a lot of kind and aware people in the world, too; I don't intend this to be an overgeneralization, but it is getting harder to ignore the rise in what seems to be self-serving attitudes circling our society these days.

Connection is on my mind as well, especially considering all that is currently occurring in the world today. Social distancing is definitely not the answer to our already-detached society. Think about how this will affect social media. If social media wasn't already a platform for the most toxic people to vent their unfounded proclamations, think about how those people are going to react under stress and even more isolation. I am thoroughly concerned about how the loss of connection, even over a short period of time, will negatively affect us and especially those of us who are newly sober and needing connection like we need air.

I am seriously considering trying to start a group of some sort for people to chat in an open and judgment-free medium about sobriety and where they can also share their struggles and successes. I don't think I have enough followers at this point to make something like that happen, but what the hell? It definitely can't hurt, can it?

I know I worry about keeping connections open and alive, so other people must feel a similar need, too. If you are reading this, please feel free to reach out any time, and I will do my best to reciprocate the gesture. I can be found on Facebook, Twitter, and Instagram all @XstopWriting. I would love to hear from you.

We are human, and we all need support, connection, and love.

Sober - Day 59

Struggling to find motivation in all this uncertainty.

We are certainly living in a bizarre and uncertain time. I traveled all weekend after receiving the news that my school is closed, and life seems to be shutting down on Friday. Today is my first real experience of not going to work, not venturing out, not living my normal day-to-day life. I have been struggling to find the motivation to write today, which is abnormal lately, and I think it is warranted to some extent. This is just not a normal day.

I learned yesterday the airlines might restrict travel domestically. This is especially concerning to me because it may affect my ability to visit my son for an unknown amount of time. This, of course, is not acceptable for me right now. I really wanted to bring my son home yesterday from California since we live in a pretty small and rural town, and neither L nor myself have to go to work. It just feels like a much better location to wait out this pandemic than Newport Beach, California, where traffic and transients are many. Nevertheless, I was unable to bring him home, so I wait and hope travel is not restricted so I can go back down to visit on Friday.

I worry about a lot of things with all that is happening around the world, but one thing is really tapping me on the shoulder and asking me to pay close attention to it. If you are like me, you have developed some new friendships with people who are newly sober and trying to make better decisions for their lives. Making the decision to be sober is difficult enough, and having to hunker down and wait out the viral storm, which has no expiration date as of yet, is not going to make anyone's sober journey any easier.

I worry about those who are not yet fully committed to sobriety. I worry about those who have not yet found their peace with their sober life. I worry about anyone struggling to make sense of all that is happening and thinking alcohol may make it just a little bit easier. I worry about anyone who does not have a support system at home to remind them \ they are doing great and they do not need a drink to feel better, calm, less stressed, or less anxious. I worry, and I don't know how to not worry about these people for whom I have now grown an affinity. They are now my people, and I would really like to find a way to reach out and help. But I can't.

All I can really do is do what I have been doing. Telling people my story and letting them know I am here for anyone who needs reassurance. Reading has been reassuring to me. Lately, I have been reading a lot. I try to always have an engaging fiction book around as well as a Quitlit book to keep me focused. Currently, I am reading *Purple Hibiscus* and, for the second time, We Are the Luckiest. When I am not reading, I am either writing my blog or my novel, which is almost halfway finished. Another way I reassure myself is by working out. It's hard for me to think about doing something toxic when I am actively promoting good health for my body. Talking to others who are experiencing what you are experiencing can be reassuring as well. There are countless mediums through which to find people who are in similar situations as us.

And, if none of this seems to be enough . . .

I just sit with the uncomfortableness of the moment and remind myself the feeling is only temporary. It will fade, and I will regain my confidence about staying sober. It sounds weird, but my therapist asked me to try doing this, and while it took me a very long time to actually trust it enough to give it a try, I am glad I finally did. It works for me. What works for you may be entirely different, but keep trying to find it; you will know when you do. It's out there, and as long as you are looking and actively taking steps to remain alcohol-free, you are winning; every single day, you are winning.

I am here for you.

SOBER - DAY 60

Health and vitality during an unhealthy time.

With the unending talk of viruses, sanitizer, health, sickness, fevers, and all manners of illness, it is difficult to stay positive and think in healthy ways about our own lives while we are stuck at home. Of course, there are two types of health we are concerned about during this pandemic. The need to stay healthy physically by distancing ourselves from others, keeping ourselves clean, not touching anything or anybody, and generally paying attention to everything that is happening around us. Then, the need to stay healthy emotionally. This is what I have been spending a lot of my time on lately. L and I are able to stay home and are not yet affected financially by this unfortunate situation, but we are both thinking about how to remain emotionally healthy and strong.

I have mentioned my coping mechanisms of reading and writing over the past two months since I quit drinking, and I cannot say enough about the positive benefits I have received from both. I was a late bloomer when it came to reading. I did not come from a reading family—quite the opposite, actually. I am pretty sure I never finished an assigned book in high school. I know, right? It wasn't until I was an adult with a teenage child that I came into reading. He was obsessed with a book, *Twilight*. Maybe you have heard of it. I decided to pick it up because I thought I should know with what he was so obsessed. Now, I need to ask for some kindness here because, remember, I was a nonreader at the time. I fell in love with the series. I devoured every book and consequently became an avid reader. In fact, I can honestly say *Twilight* was the catalyst for my going to college at the age of thirty-seven to major in literature, which I did and graduated with honors. I then went on to get my master's degree and became a language arts teacher. I have also written two books and am currently working on a third. All of this because of a silly little book that is infamous for its unreadability. I don't condone that belief, however, the book changed my life, and I will always have a soft spot in my heart for it.

Nevertheless, since then, reading has been a sanctuary of sorts for me, and I wish I could pass on my enthusiasm for reading to everyone. I was mostly a fiction reader. I tried to read self-help books but was never able to finish one until recently. I picked up *This Naked Mind*, as you all know, and devoured it, too. It was the catalyst for my decision to stay sober. I started reading it the day I quit, and I loved every page of the book. Subsequently, I then picked up, *We Are the Luckiest* and devoured it, too, and am currently reading it again because of the extent to which I relate to Laura's story. This was the book I wrote about in an earlier blog that made me break down and ugly cry in the first three pages of the introduction. Both of these books have been an incredible inspiration for me. I implore anyone who is struggling with addiction or even with life to pick up a book and give yourself a chance to find one book that changes your life forever. It's an experience you will never forget and one of which you will hang on to forever.

Writing has been part of my life for a while, too. In fact, *Twilight* is also the book that inspired me to want to start writing. Imagine that. I began writing my first book back in 2008 when Seattle was snowed in, and I was working from home. I wondered if I could write a short story. I started writing and ended up with my first book. Granted, it was not well written, but I loved the storyline. It was an apocalyptic story about negative energy taking over the world, and there were only a few people who were able to maintain their positive energy and use it to fight the negative energy. It was fun and even got published. However, it was published by a shady publishing house that later went under. I received the rights back to it, though. The second book was after I went to college and learned a little more about writing. It was a psychological thriller about a girl who was controlled by a voice in her head, and she had to find a way to overcome the power it had over her. I really love the story, and even though the writing was better, it still needed some help. Hopefully, my third book will be the charm that allows me to get something out there into the world. We will see.

My blog, on some level, has saved my life. I began writing this blog about my journey quitting alcohol the same day I quit, and I have used it to keep myself accountable every day for the past sixty days, and it has worked wonderfully. I kept thinking I would run out of things to say, and some of you probably wish I would, but I sit down to write every day, and words just fall onto the page. I feel an enormous amount of gratitude for this venture in my life, and I have loved writing about it.

Whether or not you have found your "thing" to help you feel more fulfilled and happier, especially during such dreary times, trust it is out there. Try new things, venture outside your comfort zone, and be adventurous and daring. Who knows what will turn you on to the extent your life changes for the better, forever. I promise it is worth it.

I dare you to try something new today.

Sober - Day 61

Cabin fever is beginning to set in.

My journey to sobriety did not, like many others, include the AA route with meetings, steps, and anonymity. I have heard a little about it since I quit, much of which was very positive and inspiring. Since social distancing took place this week, I have found myself feeling a little isolated at home. The beauty, however, is now that I am alcohol-free, my productivity level is through the roof. Had this social distancing occurred a little over two months ago, my life would have been entirely different. I can picture the feelings of panic about whether or not I had enough alcohol in the house; I can feel the enormous hangovers caused by day drinking on a regular basis; and I can hear the sounds of me disparaging myself because I knew it was all wrong. But, thankfully, I do not have to endure any of that because I am living sober and loving it.

While I am kicking ass in the productivity department with reading, writing, working out, and getting projects done, I do feel a small sense of cabin fever, and if there ever was a proper use for the phrase, I think we have found it. The cabin fever doesn't threaten my sobriety on any level, but the social distancing does affect my need for connection, which, as we all know, plays a large role in our sobriety process. With that in mind, I learned about an event that is taking place online through one of my new favorite authors. Laura McKowen, author of *We Are the Luckiest*, is hosting meetings online through Zoom, an online video meeting platform. I have never used Zoom, nor have I ever attended a meeting, but I decided to give it a try yesterday to see what it was all about.

I downloaded the Zoom program and signed in with a username, etc. You have to enter a meeting code and password, which you can find on Laura's website. Notice how I feel I can use her first name now; we are BFFs (I wish). Anyway, you then enter a virtual meeting room where you can see everyone who is attending the meeting and listen to whoever is speaking. The moderator, Laura, spoke about some of her experiences and then called on some people who wished to share. They shared their stories. At the end of the meeting, Laura read from her book, which made me cry; if you remember, she is the one who made me ugly cry in the introduction of her book. Well, she did it again by allowing me to hear her read her own words aloud. It was a phenomenal experience and one I would recommend to anyone looking for a connection or anyone feeling cabin fever and craving connection.

After my experience yesterday, I plan on attending her meetings daily. It is inspiring to hear people talk about their experiences. When I hear how long some people have been sober, I feel like a little baby in my sobriety. The length of my time sober does not affect the importance of what I have accomplished thus far, but it does cause me to reflect on my short amount of time doing this. I sometimes forget because I have had such a positive experience, and I feel so incredibly strong. It feels like a lifetime since I ruined my life on a daily basis at the hands of alcohol.

There is one thing of note, though, that I am feeling, and I do not know what to do with it. A lot of what I have been reading and hearing in regards to people's experience with quitting alcohol has been incredibly somber, difficult, and even excruciating. This affects me deeply because I have not had the same experiences, and being the protective person I am about people I care for, I want to help others have more positive experiences with quitting drinking and other addictions. I do not know how I can do this at this time, but I have a sincere drive to want to find a way to enact this in the near future. I hope my writing about my experiences has helped someone see a positive in all the negativity surrounding the stigma of living alcohol-free. I hope it has offered some insight into the potential for a positive experience and living a happy and sober life.

Any thoughts on how we can all better support and positively affect each other's experiences are welcome. I hope to see you at an online meeting soon.

Sober - Day 62

Mixing things up.

Being the rebel I like to think I am, I decided to mix things up during this social distancing phase of our existence. Normally, once I wake up and have my coffee, I like to write my blog entry before I do anything else. It has become an important aspect of everything I am doing in terms of accountability, so it is high on my priority list. Today, however, my rebel instincts kicked in, and I instead decided to write in my novel first. Whoa! The world was spinning for a moment, and I had to grab hold of something to avoid falling off.

I am still here, and life is still moving forward, even after my rebellious effort to alter the universe's gravitational pull on my life.

Yeah, so this social distancing thing is quite the experience. Unfortunately, for many, this is an incredibly stressful time. Employment and finances may be at risk for some. Familial and friend contact may be difficult for others. Even just maintaining homeostasis with our emotional bearing may be a struggle. Everything is just a little different in some ways and massively different in others. This is truly an important time for those of us trying to stay a course many others may not understand.

For me, staying the course has certainly not been an issue, but I have heard a lot of talking and seen a lot of writing from others who are truly struggling during this time. I feel blessed not to have those struggles right now but also cursed, in a way, because it makes me feel horrible for anyone not having an easier time. I mentioned yesterday about meetings happening around the world via platforms like Zoom for people interested in maintaining connections with their sobriety, and I think they are great. I have attended one the last two days and will continue to do so moving forward, even if only just to support those who need someone to be there.

If you cannot tell, I am struggling a little bit today with where to go with this blog because it seems there is so much emphasis surrounding the unstable aspect of our lives right now. While I continue to try and maintain a positive attitude toward it all, I wonder if anyone is listening. I don't mean to me; I mean to anything positive around us. Are we all just too distracted by everything else negative happening in the world?

Maybe it is a good time to focus on some gratitude.

I am grateful for my health and for the health of my son and my wife. I am grateful for the health of everyone who is currently remaining healthy. I am grateful for the seemingly high recovery rate from this virus. I am grateful for my family and friends. I am grateful for my newfound dedication to writing. I am grateful to have a wife with whom I enjoy being quarantined. I am grateful for the love of my son. I am grateful for my dedication to eating healthy and exercising. I am grateful for the new friends I have found on this sober journey. And, of course, I am more thankful for sobriety than anything else I have ever experienced because it is offering me the life I always knew I wanted and desperately tried to know I deserved. I now know I deserve it.

I hope all of you can take a pause and remember all of what you are thankful for as well. I have been sending out a post on Twitter every morning with five things I am grateful for. It is a good reminder of all that is good during times that don't always feel that way.

I am starting a Facebook group through my page to see if there is interest in people wanting to have a small meeting for both their sobriety and sanity during this social distancing. The group is:

https://www.facebook.com/groups/sobermilitia2020

Check it out and spread it around if you know of anyone who might be interested. I am really just starting it, so don't expect too much, yet. Thank you for all your support. I appreciate everyone who reads my blog and who likes and comments every day. You keep me going.

Sober - Day 63

Resilience and grit in sobriety.

These two words seemed to have garnered a lot of buzz over the years in regard to how they relate to business, achievement, and success. To be completely honest, I have grown tired of hearing about them because they are always being used by highly successful people who may have had experience with them on their way up, but how much resilience and grit do you need once you are at the top? That may sound a little jaded, and I don't intend for it to. I am more curious about what resilience and grit look like for the rest of us, and especially for those of us experiencing or wanting to experience sobriety. While they are similar in their roles in achieving success, they are also very different. I am no expert, of course, but here is my take, for what it is worth.

If you are reading this blog, chances are you are at least resilient on some level. You are here. You are on other sites looking into how to overcome addiction, reaching out to those who have, and hoping for some advice that clicks for you. You are reading books relating to the specific things you want to gain control over. You are taking action because you know you have a desired result in mind for the eventual outcome of your life. This is resilience, to me. There are not many people on the planet, and yes, I know there are some who just decide to give up an addiction and never look back, but the rest of us have made attempts, tried different forms of treatment, different cessation mediums, and been frustrated with our inability to quit the things we want to quit. But, when you keep coming back and looking for another way, keep asking questions, and keep looking for support, you are showing resilience every single time.

How about the times when you have begun your sober journey, and you felt as though you had it, this time. You were doing the work, making good decisions, taking the right steps, reaching out for help, and you were on your way to sobriety. Then, something happened, or nothing happened, and you slipped. You lost your strength, and you gave in to the temptation of your addiction. If you were not resilient, you would currently be even lower than you were on that day because you would have continued to fall into your addiction. But you didn't. You fell, yes, but you got back up, and you tried again. Is there anything more powerful than that? Think about how our parents told us and we tell our kids to get back on the bike, to go back out on the field, or to pick up the ball again and keep trying. We are teaching them resilience, and if we can teach it, we can live it as well, right? If you have not quit trying, you are winning every day of your life. It is when you quit, throw in the towel, and give up trying <u>that</u> you stop being resilient, and you lose the battle. None of us have lost the battle because we are here.

Now, grit, on the other hand, is a different aspect of how we approach life, problems, and addictions. Grit seems to be more inherent to me. I definitely won't say it can't be learned, but I do feel it is something we are, on some level, born with. While resilience is more of a choice, grit is either present or it is not. It sounds corny, but the phrase gritting your teeth comes to mind when I think of grit. Have you ever just hunkered down and willed yourself to do something you probably shouldn't have forced yourself to do? That feeling where you were going to make it happen no matter what. That ability to will yourself toward a singular direction is grit.

I believe the level to which we can do this is the inherent part. Some of us can do it to an unhealthy degree. I know when I was working in underwater construction, I willed myself through some shit I definitely should not have, but luckily, I came out of it alive and with all my limbs. I have consequently seen people while teaching scuba who just could not allow themselves to be comfortable breathing underwater. They could not do it. It does not mean they are not strong in other ways; it just meant they have a different threshold of what they could push themselves to do. Can this be learned? I think it can, through resilience. If we keep trying to will ourselves toward a goal, it will get easier, right? Every time we try and fail, we learn something new, and we learn we will come out of it okay, whether we succeed or not. That gives us more drive to push harder next time, more grit. Each time our grit leads us to success, we believe just a little bit more we have the strength to overcome obstacles, and our confidence grows exponentially.

What happens when we stop pushing ourselves? Do we lose grit? Does our resilience wane? I don't know about you, but I do not want to find out. If we stop trying new things, we risk not growing. Remember how when you were a kid, everything was new? Remember how each time we tried something terrifying like swimming, diving into the pool, going down a black diamond, asking someone out, trying out for a play, or going into a dark room how it took an enormous amount of encouragement and effort to make ourselves do it? But, when we finally took the leap, what happened? We wanted to do it again.

This has been a good post for me today. It has been a while since I tried something brand new. I am going to have to come up with something new to push myself toward.

Wait, what the fuck am I talking about? I just gave up alcohol and nicotine at the same time. I'm good for a little while. And so too are you. Stay the path, friends.

Sober - Day 64

Do I believe in miracles? What are miracles?

This morning while L and I sat on the sofa—her reading, me writing—she asked me a question. It was kind of out of the blue, and I had to sincerely think about it before answering. She said, "Do you believe in miracles? What is a miracle?" I looked at her, paused for a moment, then looked off into the distance for what felt like five minutes before finally responding.

We have all heard of miracles. If you were raised religiously, you have certainly heard of miracles and probably have some idea of what miracles mean to you. I was born and raised Catholic, so I had heard talk of miracles most of my life. As an adult, however, I have not even thought about the term or what it meant to me. So, when she asked me the question, I was taken aback and forced to contemplate my true feelings about what a miracle is and whether or not I believe in them.

The definition I came up with was something along these lines. A miracle is something that occurs and cannot be explained by natural or scientific methods; it is embraced by the witnesses and generally comes from a higher or divine place. Then, the question of whether or not I believe in miracles. I do believe in miracles, I have never seen one, but I believe they have and continue to happen. Then I thought, *have I seen a miracle?*

When I say I have not been a religious person as an adult, I do not mean to say I am an atheist or even agnostic. I have simply not put much energy into the idea of religion. If I am completely honest, I would say I was simply surviving over the past thirty years. I was just trying to get through the time with as little pain and heartbreak as possible. Hence the addiction to alcohol, nicotine, and others. Whatever I could find to mask the true feelings I held, I used it as a way to avoid any real truth that may have been too painful or scary to deal with at the time.

Needless to say, this stirred up some contradicting feelings within me about myself and my spirituality. After spending a little time reflecting on my ideas about miracles, I started to think maybe I have seen a miracle, and maybe I have seen one recently. If I have seen a miracle, though, I would have to concede I believe in something that came from a higher place or power, right? What does this mean about myself and my beliefs? I thought I was getting pretty close to finally figuring out who I am. Who the hell am I, then?

What is the miracle I am considering?

I am guessing you can figure it out. If you would have asked me a couple of months ago if I thought it was possible to be alcohol-free, nicotine-free, and living the life I have wanted for as long as I can remember, I would have laughed and said something like, "Yeah, I wish." Well, here I am, doing all of the above and doing them with fervor. I struggle to articulate with words adequately but continue to try, every day. Thanks for being patient while I search for ways to explain my passion for my sobriety.

Was it a miracle how I so suddenly and so easily quit using two of the most addictive substances on the planet? I don't believe I can argue it wasn't. I can say it was the right time. I can say I was ready. I can say all the planets aligned at the very moment I began this journey. Does any of this really explain what occurred to me sixty-four days ago? Nope.

If it looks like a miracle and acts like a miracle, it must be a miracle.

I don't know, but after thinking about this, thanks to L, I have to say I am at least open to the idea, which consequently forces me to be open to the idea of religion and spirituality, too, right? (Drops head into both hands and shakes head side to side.)

Sober - Day 65

"I wish you a slow recovery."

I am struggling with some feelings and emotions I am not sure what to do with at this time. Since I quit drinking sixty-five days ago, I have had a pretty amazing experience with sobriety. While there were some difficulties adjusting to new experiences with alcohol and some new ways of viewing the world to contend with, it really has been nothing but a positive experience. With that said, some things have come up for me, as of late, that have been pinging my emotional radar.

Since I have become sober, I have been reaching out into every aspect of the sober world as I can. I wanted to see what is happening out there, what people were experiencing, how people were coping, and what it looked like to everyone outside of my own personal lens. What I have found has not been as hopeful and inspiring as I would have thought. I have spoken about this a few times, but I want to expound a bit based on some new information.

Something that has been bugging me is why I have had such a positive experience with quitting alcohol and nicotine when the majority of what I see and hear out there seems to be primarily the opposite. I see and hear positive comments from those who are now sober and especially from those who have been sober for a long while. The resounding truth of the matter is for a lot of people, the process of getting sober is difficult, painful, and even excruciating at times. I have not experienced this, and it makes me nervous. Here is why.

Last night, during an online meeting, a gentleman named Sam was the guest speaker. I loved everything he had to say about his journey; he was incredibly positive and a wonderful speaker. He made me laugh, think, and appreciate where I am today. In the end, however, he said something I have not been able to get out of my mind, and I am struggling with what I need to do with this new information. He said, "I wish you all a *slow* recovery." What he meant by that is, in his experience, those who take the time to go through their process are more likely to stay the course. Some people, he says, dig in so deep they are essentially using it as a new addiction and then never really get around to the healing process.

This made me think about my journey. I have been digging pretty deep into this whole thing. I have written every single day since I became sober. I have joined groups and started going to online meetings (I had never considered a meeting before the lockdown). I am reaching out to those who ask for help, and I have started a Facebook page and now a group in the effort of giving people a place to go if they need it. Most recently, I have scheduled an unofficial online sobriety meeting for anyone who may need to share or listen to other people's journeys as a way of helping them stay on their own path. So, yeah, I am digging in pretty deep. What does this mean?

Am I replacing an addiction with an addiction? Or am I using the excess of positive energy I am now benefitting from to be a part of something bigger than my own personal goals? I mean, I am enacting every single goal I set out to achieve since going to therapy a year and a half ago. I am also doing a lot of sobriety work with others. Is it too much? I don't have any idea. I know it feels right. I know I feel stronger than I ever have. I know I am more willing than any other period in my life to help others. I just don't know how to take Sam's advice. A slow recovery.

I reached out to Annie Grace, author of *This Naked Mind*, and Laura McKowen, author of *We Are the Luckiest*, and asked them for their advice and thoughts. Annie replied it is wonderful what I am doing but I need to be mindful of self-care too. She said, "We cannot pour from an empty cup." I heard this, and I am thinking about it a lot, obviously.

Nevertheless, I do not feel my cup is empty, and I do think I am practicing self-care. However, I am now forced to consider the possibility my recovery may have some flaws in it if I am not careful. I need to be mindful the world has the capacity to take any of us down at any moment if we turn our back on it and take our sight off of the sober prize. Complacency and laziness are among our greatest adversaries as newly sober people, and it is imperative we remain mindful of our past, our goals, and our future.

Thank you for obliging me this blog to work through some of my feelings. I am going to push forward, be mindful of my self-care, and be willing to help anywhere I can. I hope you will, too.

Sober - Day 66

Stay the course.

This is the beginning of my second full week in quarantine. Yesterday was not my strongest, most positive day, but I woke up today feeling better and ready to continue down my positive and potentially too-quick road through recovery. I talked with L about my concerns yesterday, and she asked me a simple question: "Do you feel like you have recovered too quickly?" I quickly and honestly replied, "Nope." That was all I needed to hear and say to squelch that uncertainty out of my sometimes-untrustworthy thoughts. Today, I push forward and ensure above all else no matter what happens, I will stay my course.

The deeper I dig into the sober world and listen to others who are attempting to find their path to recovery and sober life, the more I hear stories of people unable to stay sober. I have been talking about this more and more lately because it is beginning to inundate my thoughts because I want to find ways to help. I am new to all this myself, and I am trying, every day, to learn some of the behavior patterns associated with quitting an addiction. I wish there was a magical day of sobriety people could strive to reach. If you make it to one hundred days, you are free and clear, but of course, there is no such day. Some people talk of quitting day to day, which means, if I just don't use today, I can worry about tomorrow, tomorrow, and then repeat. I have heard some people talk about month to month; I am just going to quit for a month and then see where I am after the month is over. That was L's mindset, originally. I have recently heard someone say they take it year to year; they decided to quit for a year at a time. All of these are different ways to approach the same goal: to quit using. Interestingly, they all have a similar underlying thread; quitting forever just seems like too much.

This, to me, is the fundamental difference between what I have experienced since becoming sober and the myriad of different stories, beliefs, and ideals I hear and see every day.

I want to be clear about something: I am not saying or even insinuating I know, even remotely, what is the best way to become or stay sober. I have a long journey ahead of me before I begin to have a true belief and understanding of this process. I am, however, trying my hardest to understand the difference between quitting easy and quitting hard. So please, bear with me.

I can certainly understand the difficulty of thinking about giving up something you love forever. It is truly a loss, something to grieve. When I quit nicotine a couple of months before alcohol, I was in that mindset. I missed it. I hated not having it. I was angry with how it made me feel. I hated how I was eating my way through it. I literally felt a longing in my soul for the thing I could no longer enjoy. It was miserable. So yes, I can certainly understand this mindset.

Here is the thing, and I am not stating any revolutionary new thinking or ideas here, but that mindset is entirely the problem. I am dying to figure out a way to write down into words how I was able to change my mindset when it came to quitting alcohol. I have not, unfortunately, figured it out yet, but I am going to keep trying because it is really fucking important.

In therapy, my therapist worked with the Cognitive Behavioral Therapy framework for my addictions. It was an idea I did not struggle to understand, but I did struggle to implement into my life and beliefs. Here is a short breakdown of the CBT framework. It starts with a core belief. For this purpose, let's say our core belief is we need alcohol to relax. I think we can all honestly relate to that one. The CBT framework suggests if we have a core belief, then we spend most of our time searching for pieces of evidence to support the belief. The core belief is so ingrained in our thinking we cannot see the pieces of evidence that do not support it. For example, there were a ton of things that relaxed me other than drinking when I was still drinking, like music, reading, movies, my dog, sex, good conversation, etc. But all of those things did not support my core belief—drinking relaxed me—so I disregarded them as a plausible solution when I felt stressed or anxious. What did support my core belief is when I chose to drink, my body relaxed, my mind checked out, and I didn't think about anything stressful.

Now, that is all fine and good, but that isn't the end of the story, is it? While those things supported my core belief and gave me a reason to justify having a drink, everything occurring after did not. For example, the hangover and continual need to drink in order to stay checked out, which, in the end, solved nothing in regard to whatever instigated the stress and anxiety in the first place. This, of course, landed me right back to square one. But it supported my core belief, so I believed it, trusted it, and was more than willing to continue following my core belief down the road and landing me here.

What CBT suggested is I needed to work on adjusting my core belief before I could begin to see all of the other pieces of evidence proving my original core belief was wrong. I had to start believing, in my core, alcohol did not relax me; it, in fact, did the opposite. Once I truly believe that then all of the prior contradicting evidence will begin to fit into my new core belief, which suggests if I am stressed, I need to put on some soothing music, talk about what is happening, and maybe read for an hour until I calm down.

There is a lot of information here, and I am sure it makes more sense to me than you because I am the one flushing it out, but there is definitely some truth to it. I know because it is how I changed my core belief about alcohol and why I am not looking at my sobriety as a period of grieving. I am looking at my sobriety as a new life, one for which I have been searching a very long time.

Tomorrow, I'll attempt to unpack this a little further as it relates to sobriety, recovery, and pretty much everything else we struggle with in our lives. It's that damn perception idea again, isn't it?

Be safe, kind, aware, and happy.

Sober - Day 67

If you are anything like me, before you quit or even if you haven't, you believed in your core alcohol was your savior when it came to feeling like yourself. It was so deeply ingrained in your psyche you could not imagine dealing with the world or people, or stress, or your family without the help of your closest friend, alcohol. Toward the end of my drinking, I was literally planning everything I did around my next drink. There was never a time when I wasn't looking forward to it, thinking about it, feeling the sadness of not having it, wondering if I could get away with doing it (when I knew I shouldn't), and generally just revering it and its place in my life. Alcohol defined my perception of myself, and it had for more years than I want to admit.

CORE BELIEF: ALCOHOL ALLOWS ME TO BE MYSELF

If we plug this into the framework I talked about yesterday, then it is pretty easy to find supporting evidence allowing us to believe this to be true. I will talk about my personal experiences but think about how it applies to yours as well.

Supporting evidence 1: I am somewhat of an introvert, so when it came time to engage in larger groups of people: parties, family gatherings, concerts, or anywhere requiring me to engage with people outside my comfort level, the very first thing I always did was find my first drink. It was almost to the point of walking into a room with blinders on and beelining it to the bar so I could get a drink in my hand as soon as possible. Speaking of which, in the last year of my drinking, one of my favorite songs was "Drink in My Hand" by Eric Church. It states, "all you gotta do is put a drink in my hand," in reference to pretty much doing anything. That was how I felt. If I had a drink in my hand, I could deal with pretty much anything.

Supporting evidence 2: I was more fun, funnier, and interesting when I drank. This was how I dealt with the above situations. If I was uncomfortable in a social setting, it was because I was insecure about my role in the setting. I was not interesting or funny; I was boring. But, once I started drinking, I was able to morph into the funny, crazy, and interesting guy everyone liked, right? That was how I saw it, and I believed it unconditionally. I never bothered to ask anyone if it were true, though. Looking back, that might have saved me a lot of heartaches, confusion, and lost friendships.

Supporting evidence 3: Confidence is the underlying emotion to this core belief. I did not feel confident in my own skin. I suffered abuse as a child, and I did not grow up in an affectionate, loving household. When my parents divorced, I was thirteen, I basically lost two years of my memory during that time for reasons I am not entirely certain. I do know I drank as much alcohol as I could and smoked as much weed as I could during that time to ensure I didn't have to emotionally deal with my life. I ended up moving out of my home and into my football coach's home for my senior year, where I did my best to barely graduate and effectively alienate myself from any friends and family I had. I immediately left home after graduation and joined the military, where I did not need to have an identity and hid under the veil of alcohol and anonymity to the point I lost all semblance of self. Then, I spent the rest of my adult life using alcohol as a way to "find" myself each and every day. In case you are wondering, I never found any part of myself while I was drinking.

New core belief: Alcohol keeps me emotionally hidden

The entire time I was using alcohol to "be myself," I was effectively ensuring I would never be nor find any part of my true self. Sure, it loosened my inhibitions, so I was more willing to talk about anything and everything, whether or not the people I was engaging with cared what I had to say. It certainly made me unaware most of the time, I was not adding anything to the conversations I was supposedly engaged in because I was not able to actually listen to anyone else's input. I was too interested in what I had to say next; I had a lot to say, and everyone cared about my opinion, or so I thought. I constantly did things I would have never done without alcohol. I remember one time I showed up to a (construction diving) job drunk because we had been called out in the middle of the night. We were in a Boston whaler fishing boat speeding out to a ship that had run aground. Our job was to save the ship from capsizing. I was so drunk while we were heading out to sea (probably about 35 knots per hour), my baseball cap flew off and I, without thinking, jumped off the back of the boat to retrieve it. Mind you, it was the middle of the night and off the coast of Oahu where I could have severely injured myself at that speed while intoxicated, and they may have never found me until morning, dead. I was a daredevil while drinking my entire life. It is truly a miracle I made it as long as I did.

Alcohol kept me emotionally hidden; it made me into someone nobody ever knew, and as it turns out, probably never liked. I can honestly and unfortunately say I have very few friends left from my days of drinking. Since it was not very long ago I finally began to find my true self, I have a very small group of close friends now.

Supporting evidence

Since I quit drinking, I have once again found my passions in life. I am living every day pursuing the things I love. I am reaching out to those with whom I want to either garner a relationship or maintain the ones I have. I am productive, active, healthy, and alive. If you meet me today, you are meeting the truest form of myself I have ever put out into the world. If you like the person you meet, let's be friends; if you don't, that is okay, too. I, for the first time, know who I am and what I deserve

Every single day I refrain from masking my true self, I find new evidence to support the belief that alcohol kept me emotionally hidden.

Sober - Day 68

One of the most profound changes I have experienced over the past two-plus months is the belief I truly deserve to be happy. It has become such a natural thought sometimes, I have to take a step back and check myself. I literally feel like I am cheating on some life examination. Why do I, after forty-eight years of feeling like I don't deserve to be happy, for good things to happen to me, to find positive relationships, or to live well, do I suddenly believe I have some worth? Thankfully, the old adage, "You can't teach an old dog new tricks," does not apply to sobriety.

Core belief: I don't deserve happiness

Supporting evidence 1: My whole life, I felt like I was simply surviving. I am not going to say I did not have positive or even wonderful things happen over the span of my life. Of course, I did. I will say this, though, any time my life began to go even remotely in a positive direction, the only thing I could focus on was waiting for the other shoe to drop. It was such a deep-seated belief I found it difficult to even feel slightly good about the things that were going well. In my mind, I held this opinion: "It was not going to last, so why try and pretend it would?" And you know what? It didn't, every single time. I thought about the negative possibilities with such conviction I virtually ensured they would happen. Do you want to know the worst part? I could walk away saying, "See, I told you that was going to happen," and not even feel upset when things fell apart. It was a self-perpetuating belief, and it worked.

Supporting evidence 2: I don't know about you, well, if you are reading this blog, I probably do, but I have a myriad of stories suggesting I was not living well back in my drinking days. Some, unfortunately, I remember very well; others, I only know the stories I have been told by those who witnessed them. Nevertheless, these stories began from a very young age for me, around twelve. That is when I discovered alcohol and when I began to collect an epic collection of reasons why I do not deserve happiness. Alcohol, as you know, erases your inhibitions and affords you the unwarranted confidence to do and say things you would not normally do or say. These brief bouts of intoxicated overconfidence generally do not end well for the practicing alcoholic. I heard a speaker at a meeting recently say something to the effect of alcohol makes things okay that are not normally okay.

Supporting evidence 3: I woke up every morning after drinking, feeling like utter shit. Unfortunately, I was doing it so often my body had become accustomed to it, and I was able to regain some semblance of vitality by the time I finished my first cup of coffee. Then, I went about my day like nothing was wrong; may I introduce to you the definition of the functional alcoholic. I never realized just how shitty I felt every day until I finally quit drinking and realized how miserable I felt while walking through life with a perpetual hangover. When you are feeling a low energy and dismal self-worth because of your drinking, you know it. You do not want to admit it, but you know why you feel worthless. Admitting it means you have to do something about it, and until you are ready, nothing sounds worse. So, you do nothing, and your energy level and self-worth spiral down until you either give up or make the decision to do something about it. In this state of mind, it is virtually impossible to feel good about yourself, your life, your decisions, or your well-being, and consequently, your self-worth plummets.

NEW CORE BELIEF: I DESERVE GOOD THINGS TO HAPPEN FOR ME

Supporting evidence 1: I quit nicotine before I quit alcohol, and it was not a pretty sight to behold. I was miserable, I gained twenty pounds, I was grouchy, and I considered many times going back to nicotine. Then, because life wasn't hard enough, I decided to add the cessation of alcohol to my to-do list. Interestingly enough, because of how my perception of alcohol changed, my perception of quitting nicotine did as well. With the confidence of quitting alcohol also came the confidence of quitting nicotine, and I haven't thought of nicotine since.

Supporting evidence 2: Giving up alcohol and nicotine forced me to make a lot of changes in my life and to view the world through an entirely different lens. My alcohol-free lens has been nothing short of astonishing. The way I now see the world has changed the way I see myself and also the way I view how and why things occur in our lives. I have taken on more positive and healthy interests during my sobriety than I ever thought I had the time for. I now have the time because I am not wasting my time on unhealthy and damaging behavior. With those positive and healthy interests come more positive and healthy occurrences in my life. The more I view my life as abundant, the more abundance seems to fill my life.

Supporting evidence 3: Okay, yes, it sounds cliche, and I would have said so a couple of months ago too, but witnessing it first-hand has changed many beliefs I have held in the past. One of the most important pieces of evidence is the awareness I do deserve to be happy. We all deserve to be happy. We just have to find a way to believe and trust that living happily will not bite us in the ass one day.

I am trying something new. I am going to try and be aware of how often I think, say, or perpetuate positivity in my daily life. The goal is to think, say, and perpetuate affirming thoughts at least 75 percent of the time.

I'll start right now. I love my sober and productive life.

Sober - Day 69

I have spent the majority of my adult life worrying about how the outside world viewed me. On some level, I guess it is important to be aware of how you are perceived by others, but all too often, people's perceptions are simply a reflection of their own insecurities, beliefs, and self-doubts. When someone goes out of their way to say something negative about you, is the comment really about you? Or are they saying it about themselves? While there are definitely times when we feel we have to say something negative, there are many other times when the only thing saying something negative does is make you feel or look negative. I am trying to listen more to my own thoughts about myself and less about others' thoughts about me. I'm going to give you two examples from my own life where I let others' thoughts of me affect my life and future.

Core belief: What others think of me matters

Supporting evidence 1: Before I even went to college and majored in literature at the age of thirty-seven, I wrote a novel. I was stuck at home during a Seattle snowstorm and thought, *what the hell, I am going to try and write something.* I ended up writing a novel. Granted, it was not well written, but I still, to this day, love the story. The novel inspired me to go to college and get my degree. I then continued on to get my master's in teaching.. While in college, I wrote a second novel. I was in love with writing, and I was trying to get better every day with the hopes of becoming a professional writer. One day, while my oldest brother was visiting, he made a comment to me that changed my life for about six years. He said, "I don't know why you keep putting stuff out there; it is clear you don't know how to write." It broke my heart, my spirit, and my drive for writing. I quit writing for six years. I cared what he said because it terrified me others felt the same way, and if they did, then that meant I must suck at writing.

Supporting evidence 2: During one of the darkest periods of my life, I taught myself how to play music in an effort to fill one of the many holes burrowing through my soul. I became pretty good at guitar, and I started writing songs (this was my first attempt at writing). The more I wrote and learned how to play, the more I fell in love with music. It became my sanctuary during a time when I felt more alone than at any other time in my life. I ended up writing five songs that I recorded myself and for which I played all the instruments, including the vocals. Granted, I was inexperienced, but I was passionate about what I was doing. I ended up trying to put a band together, and the more I engaged with other musicians, the more I learned what I was doing was not resonating with other musicians. I quit shortly thereafter. All I had to do was ask some questions, try to understand what wasn't working, practice more, and work harder, but I did not have the ability to do that because all I heard was I sucked as a musician.

New core belief: I care what I think about me

Supporting evidence 1: During both of these examples, there was one very important underlying theme affecting the outcomes: I was drinking a lot. It was my way of dealing with the pain I was experiencing during both of those periods in my life. I thoroughly believed in Hemmingway's writing motto, "Write drunk, edit sober." Alcohol was my inspiration, or so I thought. It allowed me to be more creative, or so I thought. The truth is more likely that alcohol was preventing me from having the drive to push forward through adversity, to focus clearly on my creativity, to have the patience to learn, and to avoid the distraction of negative criticism. It was far easier to just give up in my weakened state of self-worth and importance.

Supporting evidence 2: I have obviously begun to write again. This time, thankfully, it feels much different. I am writing for me. I am not worried about what others are thinking because the reason I started writing again was to hold myself accountable for my sobriety. I made a deal to write every day, and I have. Once I started writing again, I immediately remembered how much I loved it, so I also began writing another novel. I am over halfway done with my novel, and I have a goal to complete the rough draft by my birthday of April 30, 2020. My blog and my novel may not resonate with others, but they resonate with me, and I am extremely proud of what I have accomplished through writing the past couple of months. When I feel I am done with this, I will write something new. One day, when the stars align, and the energy is right, something I write will see the light of day. Nevertheless, I am writing for me, and that makes me happy.

If I am honest, I could have written for days about the supporting evidence correlating with other people's thoughts of me. It has been an ongoing disruption in my life for as long as I can remember: football, writing, music, photography, parenting, being a husband, and I could go on and on. I have always taken to heart what people thought of me because I was unable to establish my own thoughts of myself. I did not believe I held much worth, so I gained my worth from others' opinions of me.

That has and will continue to change.

If I am able to impart one single important benefit of living sober, it is this: when your mind clears, and the fog drifts away, you will begin to see yourself probably for the first time. Now, this is terrifying because everything you see after this point is new to you. You have to wade through a collage of what is your new truth and what was your old truth. You then have to discern the difference, which is the most difficult part because it takes some patience. We tend to lean toward what is familiar, and in recovery, familiarity is dangerous. We have to be able to sit in the discomfort that comes with walking away from an addiction. We have to acknowledge discomfort is present, but then we have to take its power away by not giving it any credit.

It is in this last step that your life will change forever. When you learn how to take power away from a negative belief you hold about yourself and your relationship with your addiction, you begin to see yourself and your addiction differently. You begin to see you are the person you always thought you were. You begin to believe you can do all the things you thought you could do. You begin to trust yourself, and, therefore, you begin to know yourself. This all culminates into one new core belief I have mentioned before:

You are a badass.

Sober - Day 70

I don't know why, but my sobriety days from sixty to seventy felt like a long time. Maybe it has something to do with staying home and not having as much change in my routine. Nevertheless, I am on day seventy, and I feel amazing. I'll be curious to see if I stop writing about this when I hit day one hundred as I have planned, or if I just keep letting the words fall from my thoughts and onto my and your computer screens. I guess we will see when we get there.

Core belief: I am weak

If there was one underlying belief about me when I first started therapy over a year ago that pretty much drove everything I thought was wrong with me, it would have been my belief that I was weak. What a harsh statement to hold about yourself. Was I actually weak, or was that just another misinformed perception of myself based singularly on focused data I had collected over the years? I think it was the latter, but let's look at the data I thought supported it first.

Supporting evidence 1. Well, this is obvious. I went to therapy because I was suffering from three different addictions. I had tried everything to quit them, and I did not have the strength to do it on my own. I was weak. I remember making a big deal out of breaking my vape and throwing it away after a camping trip because I had vowed to give it up before we returned home. I was ready, and I was looking forward to putting it behind me. I went home, unpacked from camping, and settled into the night before getting up the next day for work. The next morning, I woke up frantic that I did not have my vape at the ready for my first drag. My entire body revolted against me, and my mind spun out of control about how I was going to get my fix without admitting I couldn't quit. On my way to work, I bought a small vape pen, took a drag, and immediately felt better. It took me another year and a half before I gave it up for good, all the while trying to keep it from my partner. To me, that moment was the epitome of weakness.

Supporting evidence 2. For the last decade, I have at least subconsciously known alcohol was a problem for me, and I needed to figure out a way to garner some control over it. Even before therapy, I would occasionally quit for a week or even a month just to prove to myself I could do it and I was not an alcoholic. It was never very difficult because I knew there was an expiration date, so I would just grit my teeth and power through, knowing my first drink was right around the corner. It never once occurred to me to keep abstaining once my predetermined date was complete. I looked forward to that drink more than anything. As time went on and my drinking continued, I began to worry more and more about my problem. I figured if I could just not drink during the workweek, I could drink as much as I wanted on the weekends and not feel bad about it. I would make it until maybe Tuesday before caving in and having a drink. I always found some way to justify why it was acceptable for me to drink. By the end of my drinking days, I didn't go a day without a drink, and I still felt there had to be a way to moderate my drinking. There was not, and that proved I was weak.

I could go on and on about the pieces of evidence in my life that proved and supported I was weak. I could talk about my addictions, my consistent pattern of giving up on my passions, my failed relationships, my inability to maintain friendships, my feeling of worthlessness, my lack of education (at one period), my unwillingness to stand up for myself, and the list goes on and on and on. But are my failures all I have done in my life?

It is so easy to see all the failures in our lives. They hold a lot of weight because they hurt so much and so deeply when they occur. Successes are amazing too, but for whatever reason, they don't seem to stick with us in the same way failures do. If you really break it down, it does not make any sense because they should carry the same amount of weight. Failure defines what you can't yet do, and success defines what you can do. Why the disparaging weight on only one side?

New core belief: I am strong

Supporting evidence 1. Earlier, I brought up education. I graduated from high school and immediately joined the military. After four years, I got out and spent the next twenty years bouncing from job to job, trying to figure out how to survive in a world with a high school degree and not a lot of employable skills. It was a miserable existence. At the age of thirty-seven, I became fed up with my life and made the decision to go to college. I was married, with a child, working full-time, and attending college with a full load. It was one of the most difficult things I have ever accomplished, but I did it. I graduated with honors and went on to get my master's. That, for all intents and purposes, is the epitome of strength.

Supporting evidence 2. A year and a half ago, I began therapy to figure out how to overcome my addictions. I will be completely honest, and my therapist, God love her, would agree, it has not been an easy year-and-a-half road to recovery. I went through periods where I was ready to walk away and quit because things were not going the way I wanted. I uncovered dark and unsettling baggage buried deep in my core, and I went through a period where I liked myself even less than when I started therapy. It was incredibly trying, but in the end, I found my way out. I quit nicotine and then alcohol. It all came together for me, and I am currently living the life I have always wanted to live. I had a conversation with my therapist the other day about how it is difficult for me to take credit for any of my successes. I want to shower her with praise for what she has been able to help me do. But in the end, as my therapist states, I was the one who made the changes. I was the one who dug deep and found the strength to overcome my inadequacies. I was the one who discovered and accepted I am strong. The interesting part of this story was that a year ago, my therapist made a comment to me that flew right over my head at the time. She said, "I am just trying to help you see you are already a great man." There was no possible way for me to hear those words for what they were intended back then. I can now, and to my therapist, *thank you!*

Like the evidence supporting my weakness, the evidence supporting my strength goes on and on and on, too. I just had to find a way to start paying attention to it, and more importantly, to start giving myself credit for it. I have been through a lot in my lifetime, like most of you, and I spent most of my life concentrating on only the negative aspects of my life. It always comes down to perspective. How we see, what we see, who we see, and to what extent we see are always in our power. We just have to make a choice to see through the positive lens. Once we make a choice to see the positive, well, then the positive begins to flow out of us like a tidal wave. I have heard many times about how the floodgates open when we become sober. I never really understood it until now. I cry at everything, and coming from an upbringing that suggests crying is weak, it has been difficult for me to accept. But I am slowly getting there and even enjoying my new emotional self.

It means I am once again feeling; I am feeling everything, and for someone who has numbed his feelings for a couple of decades, feeling feels really good.

Sober - Day 71

Core Belief: I am unlovable

I am forty-eight years old, and I am fairly certain I have, in my past, had no idea how to properly love someone. I knew what love looked like in the world around me. I knew what love looked like in the movies and in literature. I knew what I had heard love looks like, but I honestly didn't know if I had ever truly been loved or if I had ever truly loved another human being. This sounds horribly sad, and I don't really enjoy admitting it out loud. Nevertheless, it is a feeling I have had most of my life. I know I have tried to love, and I know others have tried to love me. Unfortunately, I don't know if I have ever succeeded in loving someone or if I have ever given someone reason enough to love me.

Supporting evidence 1: I have talked about this before, but for evidence sake, I'll mention it again. My parents divorced the summer after my freshman year of high school. My dad literally threw me out of the house, and my mom was exploring the dating scene and didn't really want me around. Emotionally, I floated somewhere between orphan and homeless. I ended up living with my football coach my senior year, and some pretty weird things went down during that time in my life. From that point on, I think I have lived my life trying to validate whether or not I was lovable. I consistently came to the conclusion I was not. How could I be? To me, my parents made it clear I was not lovable. I went through high school searching for love and dismissing it even when it occurred.

Supporting evidence 2: After high school, I went through over twenty years of trying my best to find, understand, and give love. I failed on an epic level. Every. Single. Time. I am not going to take full credit for all my emotional and relational failures; I mean, it takes two and all that. But if I am honest, most of my relationships struggled because I did not understand the meaning of love. Coming from a background of emotional and physical abuse, every time I entered into a relationship, it was like a sinking ship waiting to implode. Time and again, my relationships failed. I have been married several times. I just kept trying and failing; that is all I can say to that. With each failure came validation I was simply not lovable. Somehow I feel perception is going to rear its conniving little head once again.

New core belief: I am lovable

Wandering aimlessly through life, trying to figure out what it means to love and be loved while never really seeing a concrete answer, did not help the core belief I was unlovable. How much truth really lies in that core belief? Did I never see love, or was I just unable to see love? There is a finite difference between the two. I'll also be honest there probably was love present in my life, but I just did not see or believe it.

Supporting evidence 1: My high school sweetheart. Looking back now, I can honestly say she was as in love with me as she could have been capable of at the time. I thought I was too, but after about two years, I simply broke it off. No reason to speak of, no ulterior motive, no underlying theme, I just broke up with her. I remember feeling shitty seeing how heartbroken she was, but in my experience, life just goes on after being let down. So that is what I did; I just moved on. We have reconnected as adults and talked at length about life and how we got to where we are. I have acknowledged I hurt her. She has forgiven me. We have maintained a very close friendship, and I appreciate her presence in my life.

While going through my parents' divorce and emotionally bouncing around trying to understand what love was, I had someone standing right there beside me through it all, and I just could not see it.

Supporting evidence 2: My mother. When my mom and dad divorced, my mom took off and got a place of her own.

I honestly can't remember if there was a conversation over who I was to reside with, but I ended up with my dad. He was remarried, and his wife had a son around my age, too. We lived together for a while, but I had a very difficult time at my dad's house. I won't even try to discern who was right or wrong in the scenario, but I will say it ended with my dad physically throwing me and my stereo out of the house. When I approached my mom about it, she was upset because she was living in an area that did not allow children. This, unfortunately, justified my feelings of not being lovable, and I remembered that feeling for years. But there was more. I was unable to see, at the time, my mom, knowing I had nowhere to go, left her lease and rented a new place so I could live with her. Knowing what I know now, that probably included an early termination penalty along with the first, last, and deposit for the new place. Accommodating me probably landed her in a fairly severe financial predicament. I know she did her best to be there for me, but I ended up leaving her and her place to live with my football coach because I felt unloved.

My mom was doing her best during a fairly significant life event to love and be there for me. I just could not see it. Was love present during that time? Once again, yes, it was.

If you have been following me and this blog at all, you have come to recognize I am profoundly affected by the idea of perception and how it applies to every aspect of our lives. This is especially true when it comes to sobriety and recovery. In both the pieces of evidence supporting the core belief I *am* lovable, it was always present and available for me to see, feel, and even give back. I was just not in an emotional place to see it at the time.

As I continue on my sober journey and continue to learn more about myself and those around me, I am able to see love everywhere I look. It is all around me all the time. I feel blessed I finally found a woman who is patient enough with me to allow me to find my way, even if my way isn't always the easiest way.

I now know I am lovable, my life is full of love, and even more importantly, I feel a strong desire to give love back to others.

SOBER - DAY 72

I have unintentionally enlisted in a recovery militia.

I have been talking a lot about negative self-talk and how our core beliefs shape how we see the world because it has been a huge part of my recovery process. I will continue to explore different negative core beliefs in the future, but today I decided to take a different direction for a change of pace. I also thought I would talk a little more about how my sobriety has changed my perception of not only myself but of the world as well. With that in mind, I created a small Facebook group, and we have our first official online sobriety meeting this evening. I am looking forward to seeing how and where this new endeavor takes us.

I am encouraged by the number of people the sobriety group has already garnered since it doesn't have a whole lot of activity happening yet. I hope once the group gets rolling, it will be an active place for people new and old in their sobriety to have a safe place to share and listen to stories, successes, and even failures. After all, you really can't grow without failures, too, right? One of the more interesting aspects of sobriety I have come across is the idea of relapse. There is an intensely negative stigma placed on someone who experiences this likely probability, especially in the beginning. It's probable because all of the addictions people are trying to let go of are highly addictive substances. There is a reason it is hard, and we have to take into account not everyone is going to be able to walk away clean the first time.

Here is how I look at it. Any person who has recognized they have an addiction and is actively taking steps in recovery is performing magnificently in recovery, regardless of their days of sobriety. I believe relapse can be a step in the recovery process; it may not be a step we want to take, but for some, I think it can and may be necessary. The only time I would say relapse is a negative thing is if it is followed by a person giving up their desire to change. I've said this before, but I think it is relevant enough to repeat it. While in therapy, I had reached a point of severe frustration with what I perceived as not enough growth in my quest to give up my addictions. My therapist calmed me down by pointing out one simple idea. She said, "Look at all the steps you have taken to make positive changes in your life. Do you know how many people out there are not even willing to take the first step? You are doing amazing."

That was one of the many absolutely life-changing tidbits I have come across while on my journey to sobriety and a healthier, more positive life.

A relapse can be a powerful reminder of why we are doing what we are doing. I have been talking about moderating or giving up alcohol and nicotine for the past twenty years. Both had taken over my life, and I was unable to function without either or both. I would not be exaggerating if I said I have tried to quit both at least twenty times throughout the years. Each time I was unable to quit, I eventually picked myself up and tried to at least open myself up to new ideas and approaches for getting rid of my addictions. I kept trying, and even though it took a very long time for me to finally find the one thing that pushed it all over the edge for me, I found it because I never gave up my pursuit of a better, more fulfilling life.

With all of that in mind, I have been inundated with thoughts about what has made quitting this time so much easier for me than in years past. I have been talking with other people who are experiencing the same positive experiences as well.

If there is any way I can say something, do something, or show something positive for anyone out there struggling with this absolutely horrific struggle that is addiction recovery, I am willing to try. I feel like there has to be an easier way, and I may have unintentionally enlisted myself into a life of trying to figure that out. Maybe I can call it a Recovery Militia? With any luck, some of you will be able to relate to my feelings and join me on my quest for the elusive "easy" sobriety.

Live light.

Facebook Sobriety Group: https://www.facebook.com/groups/sobermilitia2020

SOBER - DAY 73

I don't know about you, but this one stings a bit. I have noticed a lot of these negative core beliefs and thinking patterns are related in one way or another. Foundationally, however, they are very specific and isolated beliefs that are incredibly damaging. That is why I have chosen to try to break down as many as I can for you and for myself. Each time I write one of these, something new comes up for me, or I learn something new about myself and my past. It is an incredibly healing process, I must say. I hope you are getting something out of it too.

CORE BELIEF: I AM WORTHLESS WITHOUT THE APPROVAL OF OTHERS

Supporting evidence 1: I think we can all agree this is the basis for a lot of what is occurring in our world today. The social media and comment culture taking over our conscious and subconscious minds are staggering and something I do not think anyone was adequately prepared for. I know I wasn't. I remember when it all started to become a thing, I did not buy into it at all. I had my social media accounts, but I didn't really put much thought into them. A couple of years ago, however, I found myself obsessed with a new hobby, and with that hobby came the desire to put my work out into the world to see what others thought. Photography was not new to me, but I found a new passion for taking photographs. I created pages, joined groups, and started posting my photographs for all to see. The result was absolutely mind-blowing.

As the likes and positive comments began to roll in, I began to garner a sense of worth I had not known I needed. The more I posted, the more I gained likes, and the more I wanted more external validation. The likes made me feel good about myself. They drove me to do more photography and to keep posting. It wasn't until the opposite occurred I realized the danger of it all. When my posts did not receive likes, I felt depressed, unliked, unworthy. In fact, those posts that did not garner likes held more emotional weight than the ones that did. Each time a post did not succeed, by my standards, I became deeply saddened.

Supporting evidence 2: I have held a lot of passions in my life, as you have read about throughout these blogs. I have found I have been good at a lot of things, but I have never been great at any one thing. Unfortunately, there is a very specific reason for this. I have never had thick enough skin when it comes to criticism. I could hold more passion for something than anyone. I would put more work and time into it than you could believe. Then, as soon as one piece of negative criticism came in about my work, I sunk into a self-deprecating spiral of worthlessness and ultimately gave up on my passion. I wish it was not such a theme in my past, but it was, and I am fighting every day to learn how to know I am enough.

I wonder if self-worth is innate, taught, or a little bit of both? I imagine a person can learn a level of personal value as they make their way through life, but ultimately, nobody is inherently worthless. It's just not possible. We all have skills and qualities that benefit ourselves and those around us. What we learn in our life journey is not how much worth we hold but how much worth we see in ourselves. We don't learn we are worthless; we learn we feel worthless based on how we perceive the world sees us. How we feel does not equate to the reality of our true self-worth.

NEW CORE BELIEF: I AM WORTHY, REGARDLESS OF HOW OTHERS SEE ME

Supporting evidence 1: Since I quit drinking and using nicotine, my mindset has shifted in a way I never knew possible. While I understood the importance of living healthier, I never understood the damage addiction was doing to my brain. The day I quit drinking, I started writing, and I haven't looked back. Writing has always been a passion of mine, and as you know, I walked away from it for quite some time. The biggest difference I feel with my writing this time is I am doing it entirely for me. If others benefit, then that is a wonderful bonus, but I do not need the accolades or likes to propel me forward on my writing journey. I am writing because I have to write, and I am finding that to be more validating than any form of external validation I have ever received in the past.

Supporting evidence 2: I have delved into some other extracurricular activities relating to my sober journey, and they, too, have given me insight into the shift my mind has made from external to internal validation. I am writing my sober blog every day, of course, but I have also started a group on Facebook along with a writing page. Both are somewhat dedicated to the sober journey I have passionately embarked on. In these mediums, I am simply trying to make myself available to anyone who may need support or may need to just see a success story in action. I just want to be there for people. This, in and of itself, is a new direction for me. I spent much of my life simply trying to survive. I never really had time to think about service to others. With these social media platforms, I have tried to create some sober online meetings for anyone interested, and they have not, as of yet, gained traction. But here is the positive thing. In the past, had I tried to do something like this, and nobody showed up, I would have been crushed. I would have abandoned the ship immediately. The way I see it now is as long as people keep signing up, I will keep trying to be there for them. If there is no interest, then I will move on and find another avenue to try and provide a service where it is needed. I feel I have something to offer; therefore, my worth is validated by my own belief.

It took me a while, but I can honestly say the first step in my understanding of my own self-worth was my decision to quit drinking and using nicotine. By doing this, I affirmed to myself I was worth living for and I had more to offer. What an incredibly powerful sentiment for any person to hold. That is why I am doing all of this, and that is why I want to pass what I have learned on to others.

You do not need approval from others. You only need approval from yourself. Then, give yourself permission to trust you are worthy and you, too, have more to offer.

Sober - Day 74

Perception really is everything.

Those of you who have been following me and this blog for any amount of time have come to the realization I have been dumbfounded by how perception plays an enormous role in everything that has to do with recovery and change. Maybe I just missed that day in life class, or maybe I did not have the best role models surrounding positive thinking and growth mindsets. Whatever the reason, here I am, at the age of forty-eight, walking through life with a new lens that feels a little like a virtual reality headset. I am aware of every step I take forward or backward, I am aware of everything and everyone around me, I am getting a clear picture of my backstory through the heads-up display, and I feel a little off-balance because I am just not used to this new lens.

The newly sober lens is an interesting lens through which to witness the world. There are a myriad of differing opinions about its authenticity, reality, and reliability. Depending on who you talk to and what program a person used to find their sobriety, you will get an exhaustive range of emotions, beliefs, and stories about what is the *right* way to live sober. I tend to be a little bit of a rule-breaker when it comes to the way I approach life, so the idea there is a *right* way to do anything is a little annoying to me. It feels like you are trying to tell me what to do, and as my partner and I both emphatically and somewhat jokingly say to each other, "Don't tell me what to do." I bristle at the mention of a one-way approach to anything.

I have a close friend who is around the same period of time in her sobriety, and we seem to have similar views about the belief that people need to follow certain rules when it comes to quitting addictions. Recently, she posted on social media a question that was honest and pretty harmless, but she got a backlash of negative responses to it, and this bothered me tremendously. She asked what people's thoughts were on non-alcoholic wine. I quickly responded with my experiences because I have found drinking NA beer has been quite soothing, especially in times of crisis, stress, or anxiety. Unfortunately, people jumped all over her for wanting to indulge in something that feels familiar while on her sober journey. Let's not forget we are also participating in one of the biggest global pandemics we have ever experienced in our lifetime. What. The. Actual. Fuck?

One of the things I compared it to was how I have been a vegetarian for twenty years. It was a personal choice I made for a myriad of different reasons. Regardless, making the decision was not an easy one because I was born and raised a farm boy who grew up on home-raised chicken, beef, and pork. Eating meat was part of my upbringing. When I made the decision to stop eating meat, I had some changes and struggles to deal with before it became a natural reality for me to live as a vegetarian. During the process, I allowed myself to indulge in fake meat quite often because there were aspects of meat that were hard to let go of: texture, taste, consistency, etc. Fake meat allowed me to stay away from something I wanted to quit while also allowing me to get used to the idea of not having it in my life. I am now twenty years strong without the consumption of meat, and I was able to do this because I allowed myself to consume some fake meat along the way. Alcohol is no different. NA beer and NA wine have been integral in my staying sober. I don't drink NA because I secretly want to drink. There is just a comfort in the familial aspect of drinking an NA beer or having a glass of NA wine that feels comforting. It has helped me, and I am sure it has helped many of you, so why the backlash on my friend? It did not feel warranted or kind, and I wanted to write about it simply to say this:

Be kind to your fellow sobriety warriors. We are all on our own journeys here, and one person's journey may look different from another's; neither are the correct or only way to embark on this journey.

The only outcome that truly matters is staying the course with the support of our sober community. Be patient, kind, aware, and truthful in your personal journey, and remember to offer the same in regard to others' journeys as well.

PART 3
CHANGE

MY THERAPEUTIC JOURNEY

I have spoken many times throughout my blog journey about my belief easy sobriety is not only possible but probable as well. While this is not a welcomed idea in the sober community, it is what I have experienced this time around. With that said, my journey toward easy sobriety was far from easy. As you know, I began drinking at the age of twelve, and I pretty much never looked back. Sometimes, I drank before going to school. In the military, I remember drinking to the point of making myself vomit so I could drink more. I drank on the job as an adult in the construction industry. I drank at home alone for every reason or for no reason at all. I drank to feel good. I drank to feel bad. I drank because I developed an addiction and need for it to such a level it became a very large part of my identity and my life. I drank until I realized I needed to stop. Then, I drank for many more years before finding my path to easy sobriety.

Throughout my journey, I spent time with several different therapists but found only minimal success. I kept trying to use therapy because it made sense to me, even when it was not working. Finally, I found the right person with the right mindset and the right temperament to engage with for a year-and-a-half-long therapeutic journey. With her help and patience, I was able to slowly uncover and remove the myriad of layers holding me back. Then, I began to create new and more positive layers. These layers allowed me to build an emotional toolbox I could reach into whenever times or situations became difficult. Instead of reaching for a bottle to tear myself apart, I began reaching for an emotional tool to build myself back up.

You will find the extended reflection on the importance of my therapeutic journey on page 287.

BLOGS 75-101: THE ABCS OF SOBRIETY

Sober - Day 75

The ABCs of Sobriety

I have decided to try something a little new, and I am going to reach out for a little help on this one; I hope it can be both fun and enlightening. Originally, I set out to write every day for the first thirty days of my sobriety. Then, when those thirty days were over, I could not fathom the idea of not writing. So, I decided to write every day for one hundred days. I cannot believe that benchmark is now approaching, too. So far, I have been writing about my personal experiences and delved into some negative thought patterns and core beliefs that get in our way when trying to stay on our sober path. This has all garnered some positive attention, which has been wonderful to see, but here is what I want to try and do now.

I am going to write about the ABCs of sobriety and work my way through the alphabet, starting with A. I am hoping I can get some help from you along the way coming up with relevant sober words for all the letters in the alphabet. I am sure there will be a couple difficult ones. If you want to offer a word for a letter I have not written about, please comment below.

A is for Abstinence

Definition: noun; the fact or practice of restraining oneself from indulging in something, typically alcohol (dictionary.com). I always thought the detonation of the word leaned more toward sex. It turns out abstinence is literally relevant to the ABCs of sobriety.

I know it's a little too obvious, but is there really a better way to start the ABCs of sobriety than with the first thing you really need to do in order to begin your sober journey? Of course, you have to recognize you have a problem, and you have to commit to change, but your journey does not truly begin until you stop using, consuming, or performing your addictions.

I know one of my biggest obstacles with abstinence was my belief I could find a way to moderate my drinking, and yes, that might be (M) for later. But yeah, I was certain with all my addictions, well, except nicotine, I could moderate them and not have to give them up completely. In my mind, it was all a matter of grit. I thought I could will myself to follow some predetermined acceptable limit of the addictive substance or behavior. If I was successful, then that meant I was in control and able to live successfully while still using. If I am honest, I followed this belief for about twenty years, and guess what? It never worked.

I have met people who seem to be able to moderate naturally. I don't really understand it or know how to explain it, but it seems these people do exist. I tend to lean toward the belief if you are using, you are an addict, even if only to a small degree. If you continue to use, you will eventually find yourself down the path of true addiction. While this may not be fully accurate, it makes sense to me. Regardless, while there does seem to be the occasional outlier, we are just not that lucky. No matter how tirelessly we try to convince ourselves we can moderate, we just do not fall into that category of people.

After twenty years of trying to fool myself, I finally admitted and agreed I had to let it all go. All of it. Not some of it. Not some of the time. Not when it seemed damaging. All of it, all the time. It is a harsh realization to admit to yourself you cannot allow yourself to participate in something you have loved for so long, something you have leaned on to help you battle the struggles of life, and something you considered a friend. It feels like a loss and something you will certainly have to mourn. But is it truly a loss?

As you have undoubtedly witnessed me write about somewhat exhaustingly, perception is truly the major player in the success of this crucial first step in sobriety. As long as you mourn the loss, your journey will be long and painful. It is the moment that you realize alcohol is literally poison and it has no place in your body or life that you free yourself from the mourning and begin your path of "easy sobriety."

Abstinence is the practice of not poisoning ourselves. How crazy is it we don't clearly and inexplicably see alcohol as poison? If someone told you to drink gasoline, would you even consider it? If someone told you to jump off a cliff, would you ponder the possibility? If someone told you the only way to be yourself and to be happy was to inject cyanide into your veins, would you even look at the needle? No. You would not even give one moment of your thought process to consider such ridiculousness. Why? Because it is so blindly obvious all of those things will kill you.

Just like alcohol.

Sober - Day 76

The ABCs of Sobriety

A lot of what I have talked about over the past couple of months would not have ever been possible had it not been for my gaining one very critical core belief. Most of my life, I struggled to believe I had anything worthy to offer the world, my relationships, or even my family. I felt like I was an imposter everywhere I went and with whomever I found myself spending time. It is difficult to add to a relationship when you don't feel or believe you have anything to offer. It wasn't until I walked away from all the chemicals clouding my mind, spirit, and body that I began to see myself, my worth, and my place in the world. Once that began to occur, I began to believe I, too, had something to offer.

B IS FOR BELIEVE

This word has so many connotations when it comes to health and well-being and even more when it comes to addiction and sobriety. I'll focus on what I have personally experienced, and I hope you will be able to identify how it fits into your story and your recovery.

Definition: verb; to accept something as true, to feel sure of the truth of something (dictionary.com). This is an action and in my experience, a person has to have a reason to enact it in their lives. The reason can come from family, friends, partners, experiences, etc., but you cannot ever truly believe something to be true unless it comes from you.

My own internal personal belief is where I have struggled for the majority of my adult life. I did not know how to believe in myself, in my worth, in my skills, in what I had to offer, in what I was capable of, or even in who I was. I remember hearing people, coaches, friends, family say I was really good at, let's say, football, and I remember it felt good to hear it, but I never truly believed it. So, in essence, my mind and body concentrated on my personal belief about my lack of skill and only allowed myself to perform to that level. How could I push through adversity and become stronger, faster, and more precise if the entire time I was forcing myself to believe I was not capable of that kind of growth? I couldn't, and I didn't. I continued to work from a state of natural ability, which only got me so far and never took me to where I wanted to go. Want and need are certainly different emotions when it comes to making things happen, aren't they? Need means at virtually all costs, where want is basically an innate infantile feeling that instills virtually no drive. I wanted to become a great football player, but I didn't need to, and therefore, I never did.

I wrote a song over twenty years ago that spoke to my personal belief of how I would never be able to quit my addictions and, ultimately, I was going to die from them. It was a bleak song I sang and played with passion because it felt entirely true to me at the time. Think about that for a moment. Twenty years ago, I wrote a song submitting myself to the belief I was going to kill myself through my addictions. That is absolutely horrifying. What is even worse is it took me over twenty years of negative self-talk and disbelief in who I was before I finally found a way to believe in myself. Thankfully, with the help of my therapist and close friends and family, I have learned I am capable of more than I have ever thought possible. My personal work and dedication to sobriety have opened the door for me to live.

To believe in oneself is such an integral aspect of sobriety. It can be intolerably hard for us addicts because, let's face it, there are reasons we have become addicted to something that helps us escape and forget who we are. It doesn't matter how it started, who was involved, what actions we may have taken, or what anyone else thinks about us; the only thing that really matters is our own perception of our ability to believe in ourselves. I feel confident in saying each and every single one of us *does* inherently have the ability to believe in ourselves. We just have to find one thing that pushes us into our own outstretched and subconscious arms so we can first accept an inner hug and then accept ourselves for who we are. It is then we can finally begin to believe we can not only be successful and happy in our sobriety but also that we deserve to be successful and happy.

Believe in yourself; you are the only one that matters, for now.

SOBER - DAY 77

THE ABCS OF SOBRIETY

Unfortunately, today's word relates to more of my life than just sobriety, but I'll bite the bullet and try to remind myself that while I may have lived a life of perceived disappointment, I am currently living the life of my dreams or close to it, anyhow. The idea I am going to talk about is nothing new to this blog, but it is even more specific and strongly relates to sobriety. Once you abstain from alcohol, there are some other very crucial steps that can determine your level of success. One of them is today's word for C.

C IS FOR COMMITMENT

Definition: noun; the state or quality of being dedicated to a cause, activity, etc. (dictionary.com). Again, there are many ways this word relates to the topic of sobriety. It could be a commitment to yourself, to change, to your partner, to family, to friends, to your dedication to quit drinking, to your view of alcohol as the enemy, to your desire to be healthier, and on and on and on. Commitment to any major change is a crucial step because, without it, it is far too easy to talk ourselves out of our initial desire to change, as we addicts are far too aware.

For the purposes of sobriety, the most poignant attribute of commitment is in our commitment to ourselves, but I think we can incorporate a few other attributes as well. I would venture to guess anyone with whom I have come into contact via my sober journey has struggled with the idea of committing to a change. Whether it was to change a behavior or quit a substance, up until now, this has been as difficult as trying to imagine doing an Ironman triathlon. While the idea of completing an Ironman may sound empowering and validating, the reality is far outside most of our abilities to comprehend. Because of this, the majority of the world won't ever attempt one. Is it because the majority of the world is incapable of swimming a mile, biking 110 miles, and then running a marathon? No, the majority of the world could complete in an Ironman triathlon if they held one core belief: I am committed to finish.

All of us have tossed around the idea of quitting, moderating, or making a change. We knew there was something wrong with the way we were approaching our lives, but we never really took the leap. We may have dabbled in the idea of abstaining by quitting for a day, a week, or even a month just to prove to ourselves we didn't have a "problem." I remember every time I quit for a period of time how glorious it was to finally have access to the first drink again. It felt like the holy grail in my hands, and I was so grateful to once again be whole. That, my friends, is a commitment to only one thing: alcohol.

Unfortunately, that is the way society has built up social norming around alcohol. It is to be valued, praised, and even mourned when wasted. Remember the phrase we have all used when someone spilled a drink, "Alcohol abuse!" This response is taught-and-learned. Not only that, but we actually felt the sentiment when saying it. The addictive quality of alcohol is incredibly powerful, and until we admit to the power of it, we will continue to be under its power. It is when we step outside the social norming of the substance and see the absurdity of how we revere and rely on it that we can truly allow ourselves to commit to change.

For me, when I started to see the culture of alcohol for what it was, it actually became easy for me to commit to my recovery and sobriety. Annie Grace said in her book, *This Naked Mind*, alcohol is the only drug you have to make an excuse not to do. Frankly, that pissed me off. It pissed me off because I had felt the desire to lie about my quitting. It pissed me off because I had been mocked for my quitting. It pissed me off because why should anyone ever have to feel bad about making a choice toward a healthier and more fulfilling life? That one simple phrase was really the catalyst for me.

From that moment on, I committed myself to see alcohol for only what it is. A poison we systemically perpetuate as something we need in order to live a fulfilling life. I wrote earlier about how I have a very difficult time when someone tells me what to do. Well, my commitment to quit alcohol was my way of giving the middle finger to society for trying to tell me I should or need to drink.

Sorry but screw you society of alcohol.

Sober - Day 78

The ABCs of Sobriety

Today's word is interesting because it is not only relevant to the topic of sobriety, but it is also a word we have expressed most of our lives as a statement to justify why we used substances that ultimately led us to the very addiction we are discussing here today. On some level, it actually makes some sense. In order to trick our minds into thinking stupid shit is good for us, we use terminology that allows our minds to think we are actually doing something healthy, good, or worthy of our attention. It's funny, isn't it? In order to feel good about doing something we have been doing for the better part of our entire lives, we have to lie to ourselves in order to not feel like complete idiots for doing it in the first place.

D is for Deserve

Definition: verb; to be worthy of, qualified for, or have a claim to reward, punishment, or recompense (dictionary.com). We have all done things that justify our deserving of praise, and conversely, we have all done things that justify our deserving of punishment. It is an unfortunate fact of life we begin to learn as an infant and one we continue to learn throughout our adult lives. For addicts, the sentiment of doing the same thing over and over expecting different results equating to insanity hits a little too close to home, doesn't it?

I have no idea how many times, but I am certain I would be embarrassed if I did, I have exclaimed, with the utmost certainty of a man completing an impossible quest, I deserve to have a drink. My work week was so long, difficult, trying, and exhausting the very first thing I needed to do the moment I left work was to either stop at a bar, store, or at home for a drink of alcohol. I deserved it, and nobody would ever change my mind or try to argue the point with me. They would not argue because they too felt equally deserving of indulging in the tradition of consuming libations to the point of inebriation at the end of a hard day. This, of course, ultimately ends with the regret of our actions, words, memory losses, break-ups, injuries, and even physical altercations and repentant consummations. Let us not forget that while all those prospects do indeed sound enticing, even if none of them were to occur, we at least knew we were able to look forward to the coveted sickness, hangover, and physical regret resulting from our night of getting what we deserve.

Why on earth do we feel we deserve even a portion of that punishment? What did we do throughout our workweek that was so inexcusable we deserved to actively engage in our own self-punishment? It doesn't end there, though, does it? Due to our excruciating hangover the next day, we then feel the need to consume more alcohol to relieve the pain created by our initial celebratory actions. This, of course, leads to a weekend of lost time. Then, it's Monday morning, and we walk into work feeling like shit, and we wonder why we hate our jobs and our lives so much. I don't know about you, but I have come to realize I *do not* deserve to drink alcohol. No, at the end of a long, tiring, difficult, and exhausting work week, we do not deserve to destroy our minds and bodies.

It's not really rocket science, is it?

What do we deserve?

We deserve to spend a couple of days relaxing, rejuvenating, enjoying time with the people we love, and engaging in behaviors that fill our souls with feelings of worth, joy, and happiness. That is what we deserve. Alcohol and other addictive substances and behaviors never have and never will be able to replace that which we truly deserve: A life full of positivity, productivity, love, happiness, joy, friendship, passion, and peace.

How do we change our perception we deserve to be miserable to the perception we deserve to be happy? I believe it begins first and foremost with forgiveness. We have to forgive ourselves for the choices we made that set us down undesirable paths. While the addictive nature of substances like alcohol pretty much sets us up for failure the moment we begin consuming them, we have to acknowledge we did have a choice in the matter. We cannot entirely beat ourselves up for succumbing to something that is scientifically proven to be addictive, but we did play a significant role, and we have to forgive ourselves.

Once we forgive ourselves, we can ultimately believe and feel we deserve to live the life we want and then set forth with that intention.

Sober - Day 79

The ABCs of Sobriety

I struggled a little bit to come up with a word for E, but all along, I knew what I was going to write about. I struggled to commit to it because it seems to be a little bit of a controversial idea in the sober community. It's not that the idea is revolutionary or new; it just seems the idea seems to rub some people the wrong way. If you are one of those people, I apologize in advance and ask you to try and understand this is only my perspective, and while it may not resonate with you, it may resonate with someone else.

E is for Easy

Definition: adjective; achieved without great effort; presenting few difficulties (dictionary.com). The word easy contrasts highly with the word addiction in general but even more so with the idea of letting go of an addiction. Our entire lives, we have heard people talk about how difficult it is to change. We have been told in times of change to simply "grin and bear it." I know I have certainly experienced such feelings toward my addictions in the past. I remember feeling like I was literally just gritting my teeth and forcing myself not to drink, smoke, etc. It is an awful feeling and one I do not wish to ever experience again.

If you have been following this blog at all, you know I have been touting the idea of easy sobriety for quite some time. At the beginning of my sobriety, I was not aware my experience was so different from others because I did not follow the more traditional routes of recovery. I had considered using programs several times over the past twenty years, and I would say I probably even googled it a couple of times while trying to find my own way. The only true experience I had to draw from was my partner's, who quit thirteen days before me, and mine. Since we have had very similar experiences, I figured it was not uncommon. I was certainly aware of the difficulties in quitting addictions because only a couple of months prior, I had quit nicotine, and that was a disaster of an experience. I'll come back to this later.

Once I began writing about my experience, I also began reaching out to some people and groups, including some online sober meetings. It was truly an enlightening experience and one that has propelled me on a side journey I never expected to find myself on. What I learned was there is an enormous group of our sober brothers and sisters out there who have had a terrifyingly difficult time quitting their addictions. I felt this to my core, and it has inspired me to want to learn more, to experience more, and to figure out the difference between hard and easy sobriety.

That is the bottom line for me, and I hope it is for some of you as well because it changed my entire life. When we make a major change like quitting an addiction, we see it as something to mourn, and based on our relationship with the addiction, it feels right to us. We are losing something we love, so why shouldn't we mourn it? That dilemma, to me, is the essence of hard sobriety. When I read *This Naked Mind* by Annie Grace, I made an immediate shift in my relationship with alcohol. I went from loving it to feeling severe contention with everything about it and especially the societal normalization of it. I could no longer stand to hear comments like, "I deserve a drink," or "Don't spill it; that's alcohol abuse," or the now ever-popular "Quarantini" trend that is catching on. I just had no use for any of it anymore, and subsequently, my "mourning period" lasted about a day, and that was truly the end of it. On top of that, another unexpected benefit emerged from this way of thinking that consequently lessened my desire for nicotine as well. Every day since I have experienced continuous growth in my awareness of something that is globally recognized as a "need" while simultaneously suppressing and even killing us. I just don't miss it at all.

I know there is no one right answer for everyone, especially with regard to addiction and recovery. I know we all have to find our own way and experience for ourselves what works in changing our relationships with our addictions. I also know, for some, religion is a major component in this battle for sobriety, and that is perfectly okay, too. I think the major takeaway in regard to trying to understand the difference between hard and easy sobriety is as simple as the answer to this one question:

On a scale of 1–10 (with 10 being the most positive), how much do you rate alcohol's contribution as it pertains to your personal and social well-being? If you chose a high number, you are probably viewing alcohol as something that relaxes you, it allows you to be yourself, it gives you the courage to do things you couldn't otherwise do, it makes you more creative, it allows you to be more social, and make more friends, etc. All of which are false beliefs we have learned from a very young age through a more exhaustive effort of marketing and social normalizing than any other product in the history of our planet. Nothing is publicized, broadcasted, and published as "socially and personally beneficial" as much as alcohol. There is a reason for that.

I searched for and found reasons to knock my number down to 1 and even 0. I now believe alcohol has no positive contribution to any aspect of my life.

And so, it doesn't.

Sober - Day 80

The ABCs of Sobriety

There is no question whatsoever what the word of the day for F has to be (no, it's not that). It's probably the most quintessential piece of sobriety and recovery. I know for me it took a long time to find it or to even find a reason why I deserved it, but in the end, it was not until I allowed myself to receive it I truly began to recover and begin my new life of sobriety.

F is for Forgive(ness)

Definition: verb; to grant a pardon for or remission of (an offense, debt, etc...); to absolve (dictionary.com). This word is almost entirely about wrongdoing on the part of the user. As addicts, there is not a single one of us who has not committed some offense while using we regret or for which we paid some high price. It's part of the deal, isn't it? Alcohol alters our mind and consciousness; we do not think clearly, we have fewer inhibitions, and therefore we do stupid shit. Then, almost immediately, once we regain full consciousness, we feel bad for what we have done. For some of us, this may have become a daily/nightly routine. For others, this may have only occurred a few times. Regardless, for all of us, there is at least one time we all remember that truly tipped our needing-to-quit scale into the full on position. Hence, all of our presence here.

It is easy to see how forgiveness plays a critical role in a person's recovery and ultimate sobriety. Everyone who has been close to an addict has had to let things hurtful slide simply because they loved the person who made the inebriated mistakes. For the addict, recognizing these things and owning up to them is literally a step in the process for some of the abstinence programs. We have to make amends, make wrongs right, and fix the things we screwed up. In the process, we have to be aware the affected people may or may not accept our apologies, and they may or may not forgive us as well. In order to heal and move on to the next step in any program's progression, we have to understand the unfortunate potential is there, and we have to be able to accept it. It is not the affected person's responsibility to make us whole again; it is ours.

While forgiveness is a well-known and understood fact of successful sobriety, I believe the other side of forgiveness is even more important. I believe this because unless the offender truly forgives themselves, I don't know if it is possible to even begin accepting forgiveness from others. Taking this to another level, I don't think a person who has not forgiven themselves can even begin to ask for forgiveness in the first place. Simply asking for forgiveness is easy. We can do it even if we don't believe we deserve it. Forgiving ourselves is hard; incredibly hard. It is hard because we, more than anyone, know what we have done. Not that we may even remember the event, but because we know ourselves while using, and we know we are capable of doing most anything someone tells us. We have become accustomed to hearing the stories. The more we hear about the stupid things we have done, the more we believe we are incapable of change and unworthy of forgiveness. The longer this goes on, the more deep-seated those feelings become.

How then, knowing what we know about ourselves, can we ever get to a place where we are capable and willing to forgive ourselves? The first step is to truly acknowledge we are human, and every person from whom we are seeking forgiveness has made mistakes. Granted, ours may carry more turbulence, but we are nevertheless all human. Then, we have to understand, accept, and believe our addictions are not entirely our fault. I know this is a victim mentality, but there is scientifically proven data to support it. I struggled with placing blame anywhere but on my own shoulders, too, and I came from an abusive background; I just had a hard time saying someone else was responsible for my bad decisions. However, it is becoming a somewhat-accepted viewpoint because of alcohol's incredibly addictive qualities, if a person drinks, they are susceptible to alcoholism. The only variable is the amount of time it takes someone to become truly dependent on it in their daily lives.

Now, even though I have come to believe this to be true, I also feel, in any research or data, there are always outliers. Regardless, the outliers are few and far between, and I think it is time for all of us to let go of the alcoholic stigma of being the problem and accept the fact alcohol is the real problem and we really are victims of its addictive chemical makeup.

Here is the catch.

We are only allowed to feel this way one time. The moment we understand the addictive nature of alcohol and why it has had a negative effect on our lives is the moment we need to begin taking responsibility and making the necessary changes to remove it from our life. We have, in effect, evolved, and we are no longer able to use the excuse of ignorance to justify our behavior, not that we ever really could have, but you know what I mean. It is in this evolved state we can accept what occurred in our past, learn from our mistakes, understand we are worthy, and then forgive ourselves for whatever we have done with the following caveat: we will work toward recovery and live a life of sobriety.

We may never receive the forgiveness we seek from some people, but we can at least know we have taken the necessary steps to do all we can do. We do not have to look back at our past and feel as though we could have done more or tried harder. Hopefully, with all we have learned along the way, we have recognized the behaviors that are unforgivable, and because we have evolved, we can rest assured we will never again allow ourselves to be in a position to seek that kind of forgiveness.

I've said this before, but my cousin attributes her success in life to one simple life attribute:

Living well.

Sober - Day 81

The ABCs of Sobriety

I really thought the ABCs of Sobriety were going to be more difficult to come up with, but each day, a new word is just waiting to be written about. I told my therapist this yesterday, and she laughed at me. When I asked why she was laughing, she responded how differently my thought patterns are from only a couple of months ago. I would have never said something like, "F is for forgiveness, because, I mean it has to be, right? You can't be sober without it." It tickled her, and in return, it made me feel good because I like surprising the person who has been there throughout my otherwise tumultuous therapeutic journey.

G is for Gratitude

Definition: noun; a feeling of thankfulness or appreciation, as for gifts or favors (dictionary.com). Holy shit, how much do we have to be grateful for as people in general? Let alone those of us actively engaging in sobriety? This word is loaded with so many levels and layers, I don't even know where to start.

Gratitude. I, unfortunately, think this word is slowly losing some of its potency for people and as a society. I can say this because I know, before becoming sober, I was not actively engaged in showing gratitude for much of anything. I was able to recognize good things when they happened, but I looked at them as more of a coincidental occurrence rather than an intentional or purposeful one. I took care of the things important to me because I knew they mattered for my happiness or wholeness as a person, but I never felt gratitude for them. They were just there, and I did the best I could with what I had around me.

Since I quit drinking, I have begun a few routines to help me remember to show gratitude every day. One routine I have adopted is to post on Twitter a list of five things I am grateful for every day. It sounds silly because I had never been a Twitter person, but I have been engaging with it as a way of trying to support some of my writing, my Facebook sobriety group, and my online meetings. The way my post looks is like this, and I will post this simultaneously as I write this blog:

I am #Grateful for 1. My son's positive growth into a young man. 2. Being "stuck" with two of my favorite people. 3. My dedication to pursuing my goals and passions. 4. My #sobriety. 5. Later today, when I take my 392 SRT Challenger out for a drive.

I just posted it. The point is, I am actively trying to practice the art of showing gratitude every single day. While it may seem like a silly way to do it, it has helped me remember to stick to the plan.

Coincidentally, I just talked with L and X yesterday about wanting to reread and watch *The Secret* again. I read it about seven years ago. It resonated with me tremendously, but I was in no way ready emotionally or mentally to try and enact its lessons into my daily life. I told my therapist last night I am now ready. Her face beamed from my statement because she is a strong proponent of *The Secret*, as well, and especially as it correlates with the CBT framework I talked about earlier. The fact I now believe I am ready to try and incorporate *The Secret* into my life shows I now believe in my worth, my capabilities, and my deserving of a better life.

I believe all of my new beliefs about myself are a direct result of the gratitude I feel for my sobriety and for the amazing and abundant life that is now unfolding before me. I see the love from L every day. I see my love for her. I see the endless potential in my son. I see the wonderful and blessed life we live. I see the perfect health we are all blessed with, and I see the way we intentionally take care of and protect it. I see a future full of adventure, success, and happiness. I see things differently now because I have allowed my eyes to open and to take in all the abundance that is around my family and me every single day. I believe there is nothing but abundance out there for us.

This positivity has never before been a part of my vocabulary, but it is now because I am grateful for everything and everyone around me every day. I may be the most blessed person on the planet. However, that can't be true because each and every one of us is the most blessed person on the planet. As long as we can all continue to allow ourselves to see and believe it, then it is true for all of us.

Be grateful.

SOBER - DAY 82

THE ABCS OF SOBRIETY

I woke up this morning to another sunny day in Washington state and a forecast of ten days of continuous sunshine. It is April, right? April showers and all that. That phrase, I am pretty sure, was coined in the Pacific Northwest. I'll take it, and I'll take it with a smile while taking a walk, washing my car, and probably mowing the lawn, too. I love Washington state in the sunshine. If you have never been here, it's a pretty magical place with all the greenery for which the emerald city is tagged. Anyway, back to writing about the forever-evolving and interpersonally constructed world of sobriety. I have always thought about writing a blog, but I never thought I had enough to say about anything; well, I found my thing for which to write about. Today's word has two plausible meanings, both of which I find to be incredibly relevant to the idea of sobriety.

H IS FOR HEALTH

Definition: noun; the general condition of the body and mind with reference to soundness and vigor (dictionary.com). The word *health* came to mind almost immediately when I sat down to write the word of the day for the ABCs this morning. Interestingly, for some reason, I struggled with it because I was only grasping the idea of physical health, and that is not always the most motivating angle for some people. On a whim, I decided to look into it more deeply to see what the internet had to say about it. Of course, every thing I could find referenced both the body and the mind which resonated strongly with me, and I hope it does with you as well.

The body. If you have been drinking steadily for any amount of time, you have undoubtedly noticed a downward trend in your physical health. The most damaging aspect of this negative consequence of drinking is its slow downward trend. You don't really see or feel it happening until one day, years down the road, you get up one morning and look at yourself in the mirror to find a fragment of the person you once were. You see bloodshot eyes, a drawn and reddened face, wrinkles, blotchy skin, and a sadness you don't remember garnering over the years but feel, nonetheless. You may have lost your young physique you once had due to a lack of motivation to work out every day or even a couple of times a week. Your head aches, and you can't think about anything but how to make it stop. You think about having a drink because you think it will help you feel better. You even know it will only give you the illusion of feeling better, and that is okay with you. You don't because you have to go to work, or you do regardless, just to make the pain go away. In the end, after years of battling with yourself about the potential need to stop drinking, you finally give it a try and are astonished by the results.

Your skin clears up, you begin to lose weight, your eyes clear and have more depth, you wake up refreshed from a good night's sleep, you look happy and healthy, your friends comment on how much younger you look, you feel strong and confident, and you ask yourself every day, "What the fuck was I doing to myself for all of those years?" The answer is quite simple, really. You were poisoning yourself because society not only told you to but because they assured you your life would be so much better if you were drinking.

It was a lie.

The mind. The body is one thing, and yes, it is the vessel that carries the mind. Nevertheless, the mental gain from quitting drinking has been the most astonishing revelation and benefit for which I could have ever hoped. While I was drinking, I held very little focus, drive, care, or passion because I was always a little emotionally off. My mind was always fighting to remember things, my head always hurt, my body felt tired, and I could not, for the life of me, find a reason to work hard at anything. It was not all that long ago, but I can honestly say I cannot believe just how lazy and unproductive I had become. I was a functional alcoholic, which, to be honest, is a curse. It gives you the illusion you don't have a problem because you are getting through life, making money, and providing for yourself and your family. There is no blindingly obvious reason to second-guess yourself.

From the day I quit drinking and from the perspective from which I did, my entire life began to change. My physical body quickly came around and thanked me for my positive actions. My mindset, however, is truly the thing I cannot get over. While drinking, I tiptoed through life feeling unworthy, insecure, and unable to do or be anything other than what life had shown me. Or, I should say, what I perceived life had shown me. Through a clear and present mind, I have begun to see a world I have never seen before. I am truly seeing a world filled with potential and possibilities, a world filled with love and good people, a world open and ready to listen to what I have to say, and a world patient with me while I found my place within it.

There is no way to adequately express the gratitude I feel for my current mental and physical well-being. I am actively pursuing my goals, passions, and even a need to be of service to others. I want to help, I want to learn, I want to grow, and I want to live, and you can, too.

That is no lie.

SOBER - DAY 83

THE ABCS OF SOBRIETY

When I look back over the past forty-eight years of my life, there is one common thread I see running throughout all of my life's journeys, accomplishments, failures, and even hopes. This thread is the foundation for what has kept me stagnant, unmotivated, uninspired, and void of commitment. I was never taught it was important in our day-to-day lives. I did not understand a person needed to actively engage with the "letter of the day" to succeed in life. I can say, looking back, I saw it throughout my life's journey; I saw people living with it, but I just could not conceptualize how to bring it into my otherwise unintentional life.

I IS FOR INTENTION

Definition: a determination to act in a certain way; resolve (dictionary.com). I really love the last part of this definition. The first part, having the determination to act in a certain way, makes sense and aligns with what I would have said if asked for a definition. It's the last part that resonated with me more in regard to how it correlates with sobriety. Resolve. I love it.

Let's start with the word itself; intention. Ever since I met L, I heard her speak of intention. She would say things like, "I have to set my intentions for the day," or "That is not part of my intentions." I've heard her. I even kind of understood her, but I had never met anyone who actively set intentions for a day, week, month, or year. I couldn't comprehend it fully, so I disregarded it, frankly. It was nothing against her; I have always looked up to her as a successful and strong woman, but the way she achieved her success was extremely foreign to me. It is interesting to be surrounded by exactly the energy, potential, and motivation you need before you are actually ready to receive, use, or even understand it.

Once I finally made the elusive decision to quit drinking and live a sober life, everything began to change and it changed rapidly. I unintentionally began to set intentions for myself, my life, and my way of living. I set goals to read more, write more, exercise more, and be more productive in general. All of these things, from the day I quit, I have enacted, and I am witnessing a change in the way I experience the world every day. Living with intention offers a fulfillment I have never before known. My days are filled with successes (and failures), ideas, and abundance. With each new goal I set and achieve, I feel more confident. With each new idea I try, I feel more creative. With each day I exercise, I feel healthier. With each book I read, I feel more enlightened. Every day brings forth new and exciting experiences, learning, joy, happiness, love, and life. For the first time in my life, I understand the sentiment of there not being enough time in the day.

Now, let's look at the last part of the definition. Setting intentions for the day has caused me to actively engage with not only the world but with my world. I am actively participating in the way my life plays out. I am encouraging results, I am clearcutting paths for me to follow, and I am making myself available and open to people with whom I share commonalities. I am writing the script of my life every day I wake up and decide, by setting intentions, to actively play the leading role in my story. The resolve aspect of intention is the end result, and you have every ounce of power to control the outcome.

How does this affect the addict?

What is every single one of us who are joining sober communities, attending meetings, or downloading sober apps trying to do? We are trying to fix something we feel is broken, missing, or forgotten. We are trying to make a positive change in our lives. We are trying to resolve the past and roll out a new and more fulfilling future. We are able to do this by setting intentions for our mornings, afternoons, evenings, days, weeks, months, years, and ultimately lives.

With each intention we set and achieve, we resolve something. We resolve an aspect of our past and open doors to new paths, new options, new experiences, and new lives. We hold the key, the power, and the will; we just have to choose to live with intention.

What is your intention for the day?

Sober - Day 84

The ABCs of Sobriety

The letter of the day today was not the easiest, and as you may have already seen, I kind of like to play on the not-so-obvious meaning of words when I can. Joy came to mind immediately, but for some reason, it did not resonate with me in regard to sobriety. I, of course, have felt more joy now than at any other time in my history, so it is relevant, but it just wasn't the direction I wanted to go. Interestingly enough, the word I kept leaning toward and kept coming back to is one with meanings, making it a very flexible word in our vocabulary.

J IS FOR JUST

Definition: adjective; acting or being in conformity with what is morally upright or good (dictionary.com). We use this word for so many things, and I was not aware of the flexibility until I really looked at the way we use it in our language. It can refer to direction: it's *just* over there. It can refer to precision: it was *just* the right amount. It can refer to minimally: it was *just* last week. Or it can refer to a lot: it was *just* wonderful. If you enjoy the meaning of words, the more you look at this word, the more your interest may pique, especially in the way we use it. For people living in sobriety, the word "*just*" just might be the word we are looking for, but not for the meanings stated above.

When using the actual definition stated above, my mind immediately begins to wander down the path of the addict's mindset and asks why he or she began using in the first place. For me, my addictions certainly stemmed from my inability to live or feel worthy of a *just* life. Before I try to define what a *just* life might look like, let's look at what an un*just* life looks like. You know, the life we all lived before finally finding the elusive reason or reasons to become sober. My drinking, nicotine use, and other addictions kept me from ever seeing my true self. It kept me down, depressed, and feeling unworthy of living a fulfilling life. I was certain I had come as far as I could come, and settling into my unfulfilling life was the only way to save any semblance of my sanity. I mean, why fight the inevitable? I was destined to live an un*just* life. Believing I was deserving of unhappiness, I never had the chance to see from another vantage point. I only had one lens, and it was a lens of dejection.

Quitting alcohol, nicotine, and other self-deprecating addictions and behaviors afforded me the ability to finally see through another lens, and the lens was a lens of *just* happiness. Why is the new lens of happiness *just*? Because all of our lives begin with a *just* beginning as babies. We are all born deserving of feeling love, happiness, joy, silliness, to be fed, cared for, sheltered, and any other humane traits you can think of. We all deserved it because life is meant to be *just* for everyone. As humans trudging through the chaos of life, we are bound to make mistakes. Some mistakes are small, some big, but all are, to some degree, expected. Those mistakes do not negate the fact we are all deserving of a *just* life.

However, we must be able to see, believe, and understand we deserve to live in a *just* world intended for everyone. However, as long as we suppress our minds, bodies, and spirits with the use of addictive chemicals and behaviors, we will not be able to accept that we are worthy of a *just* life. Therefore, we continue to trudge down the path of the un*just* life we chose for ourselves. Unfortunately, like many aspects of sobriety, it is all up to us to make the choices separating the easy sobriety from the hard sobriety and the good life from the bad life. "Choice" should have been my C-word because, ultimately, it all comes down to whether or not we choose to be sober, choose to be happy, choose to be successful, and choose to live.

It is no state's secret our happiness is really up to us. I know, at times, it seems like the world may be conspiring against us, plotting to take away every easy path, creating constant obstacles to overcome, and generally making our lives feel like a junkyard of trash from which it is impossible to emerge victoriously. Remember, though, the pile of trash we may currently find ourselves standing in may only be our perception. If we change our perception, we may afford ourselves the ability to see the trash we have envisioned standing in is, in fact, actually a pile of jewels.

We *just* have to believe we deserve and are worthy of living a *just* life.

Sober - Day 85

The ABCs of Sobriety

For those of you who do not yet know, I am a teacher by trade. I work with special education for junior high school students in the area of language arts. One of the non-negotiables in my classroom revolves around today's word. It is something that has always felt important to me, even before I began to fully see and understand my own personal growth and potential in this area. In a world seeming to lean more toward a selfish, self-absorbed, self-centered, and narcissistic ideology, I feel like we are losing sight of others in regard to empathy, awareness, and general caring for those with whom we come into contact. During this pandemic, in-person contact is not as easy and often, but contact via online mediums is at an all-time high. While it does not seem as personal, the effects of negative online interactions may have the same or even greater impact on a person.

K is for Kindness

Definition: noun; the quality of being friendly, generous, and considerate (dictionary.com). The root word, kind, also means being affectionate or loving. If we, as a society, allow ourselves to slip into a realm of narcissism, we risk losing the ability to act kindly toward others. We can be kind to ourselves, which is what I worry about in terms of how kindness relates to sobriety because if we lose our ability to be kind to others, could we then also lose the ability to be kind to ourselves? It's actually quite a terrifying prospect if you take a moment to think about the possible ramifications.

I believe it is safe to say anyone suffering from any addiction also suffers from an inability to treat themselves with kindness. I mean, if you were kind to yourself, would you really actively participate in poisoning yourself? No. Would you actively participate in behavior causing you to feel depressed, unworthy, unmotivated, or unlovable? No. Would you go out of your way to put yourself in a position to virtually ensure you will lose all semblance of self? No. The only reason anyone would do this is they do not believe they are deserving of consideration, love, generosity, affection, or friendship. You cannot be kind to yourself if you do not feel worthy of the connotations of the word.

If you cannot be kind to yourself, is it truly possible to be kind to others? This is a little bit of a contentious thought because most of us do not want to admit the answer may be no. Even while using, some of us may want to cling on to the idea we were still good and kind people. But, what if we were not? What would it mean about us and our relationship to the world? It could mean we were bad people, and that is a pretty awful realization for anyone to come to. What if, instead, we said while using, we did not always act from a place of kindness, even though we know in our heart we still held the ability to do so? Would it sting less? Probably, but let's not focus on the negative because, let's face it, we all did unkind things while using. Those actions are most likely what led us to become sober, sober curious, or trying to get sober.

Let me tell you a little bit about what I have noticed about kindness while traversing my sober path. Before finally making the decision to quit drinking, I can honestly say I thought mostly about myself. I loved my wife, my son, my family, and friends, of course, but if I was to truly consider where I spent most of my energy, it was in regard to my own needs. At the end of my drinking days, I was thinking about my first drink by the time I had my first cup of coffee. From then, the trajectory of my day revolved around getting to the point when I could drink. If it was a weekend, then it was immediately after my first coffee. I thought about nicotine and whether I had enough to get through the day. I thought a lot about when I could get my next fix because I was still using it even after I told my family I would stop. I would make up reasons to get away so I could use it. I had addictive behaviors negatively affecting my relationships with people. Basically, I was living for me and my next fix of whatever I happened to need at the moment. Did I still love the people around me and do my best to take care of them? Of course, I did, but did I do it to the best of my ability? I did not.

Since becoming sober, my view of the world and the people within it have changed dramatically. I honestly don't know how to keep up with or have enough time to do all the things I want to do for others. I have set a lot of goals for myself, and I am scheduling my days to ensure I am completing those goals. I am also ensuring I have enough time to do all of the other things in life I have missed out on over the past thirty or more years I wasted while using. I have played with my ten-year-old more in the past couple of months than I ever did before. I am doing things with him and my wife they love just so I can spend time with them. I am able to articulate my feelings better than before. I am able to resolve conflicts with a much better temperament than I knew I was capable of. I spend more time tucking in my son. I spend more time conversing with my wife. I remember to check-in when I see she is struggling. I remember to do all the things I did when we first met. I am able to do all these things because I am not distracted by my own selfish needs.

Sobriety has afforded me a life I always knew I wanted but never knew I deserved. I know in the deepest part of my soul I am a better dad, a better husband, and a better person. I know this because I am now acting from a place of kindness to myself and to the people around me.

Be kind, not because you should be, but because you can't help it.

Sober - Day 86

The ABCs of Sobriety

It's Easter Sunday, and while the obvious "L" word of the day is probably love, I think there is a word that is even more relevant to sobriety. I am willing to wager a handsome sum every single one of us who are reading this blog, joining sober groups, attending meetings, and seeking help have felt, at some point in our lives, we have struggled to do the word of the day or at least struggled to do it well. Fortunately, if you are here reading this blog, joining sober groups, and attending meetings, you are, at the very least, beginning to take the necessary steps to give yourself the opportunity to start doing it fully. Congratulations!

L is for Live

Definition: verb; to have life, as an organism; be alive, be capable of vital functions (dictionary.com). In order to fully understand the meaning of today's word, let's also look at the root word, life. One definition is as follows: noun; the power of adaptation to the environment through changes originating internally (dictionary.com). To live a life could simply mean not to die. But, to live a life worth living and one we are proud of is an entirely different ideal. It is an ideal I never really knew existed growing up or while I trudged through adulthood. I just figured we had to do what our elementary teachers taught us, "We get what we get, and we don't throw a fit." That's what I did for the better part of thirty-plus years. I just lived life as it came to me.

The first and hardest step in living well is to realize and accept that we were not simply victims while we were using. We were active participants in the slow and intentional disintegration of our lives. As long as we believe we played no part in the outcome of our lives, we cannot take steps toward making the changes necessary to live the life we all inherently deserve. Once we see, accept, and begin acting as role players in our lives, we then have the power to see how things can be different. And the difference is overwhelming.

Now, the really interesting, and quite frankly, fucking amazing facet of this whole idea of living life is the fact there is no single right answer to what it means. Every single person holds the key to their own definition of life and what it means to live a happy, productive, and successful one. It is up to us to discern what living life means to us, individually. How cool is that? We can literally write the definition of the words live and life based on our own beliefs, experiences, and desires. If you are not jumping up and down right now (virtually), high-fiving everyone around you, and singing "It's My Life" by Bon Jovi, I don't know what to tell you. Take hold of the reins and start writing your own narrative.

After looking back and regretting the past thirty-plus years of my life, I am developing a pretty serious personal belief and comprehension of what it means to live. While I honestly don't believe I missed all of those years, I am one hundred percent certain I could have done a much better job of living. Here is my working definition of what it means to live a good life. I wake up every morning and give thanks (not to God but to the universe) for the life I live. I give thanks for my son, my wife, my house, car, and job. I give thanks for the love, joy, and happiness surrounding me every day. I give thanks to my friends and extended family. I give thanks for my and my family's health, especially during these times. Then, I set intentions for the day. I decide what I will walk into the day believing and doing, and then I do it. My intentions look something like this:

1. I am a great father and husband. 2. I am a professional writer. 3. I act from a place of kindness. 4. I write in my novel. 5. I write my sober blog. 6. I exercise every day. 7. I give and allow myself to receive love. 8. I am the best version of myself.

I try to write my intentions from a perspective of who I am and what I am doing rather than what I want to be or do. I believe those things are already done, and I remind myself every day. Once my intentions are set, I approach my day with the greatest amount of positivity I can. If I feel myself begin to drift toward negative thoughts or beliefs, I try and catch it and remind myself of the things I am grateful for. This, generally, cheers me back up, and I can continue my day with positivity. It may not always work, but I believe the more times I make it happen, the easier it will be each time I try. The rest of my day, I work toward completing the goals I have set and loving the people I am with.

I live each day with passion, intention, and love in my heart for myself, my family, and my fellow persons. I have lived more in the past eighty-six days than I think I have in the past forty-eight years of my life. It's never too late to begin living the life you never knew you wanted or deserved.

SOBER - DAY 87

THE ABCS OF SOBRIETY

Today's letter and word is certainly a tough one because we have all needed, if not begged for it, at some point throughout our sober journeys. In order to carry a burden heavy enough to require one to request, beg, or plead for it, a person has had to suffer a great deal of physical, emotional, and personal misery. We have had to feel we cannot obtain it on our own. It is an unfortunate characteristic of the consequences stemming from the inevitable loss of one's self on the way down to our bottom. Much like yesterday's word, the definition of one's bottom is defined and created by us and us alone. Nobody took us by the hand and led us down to our bottom. In fact, it can be argued we made that trip all by ourselves, and we made it willingly.

M is for Mercy

Definition: noun; compassion or forgiveness that is shown to someone whom it is within one's power to punish or harm (dictionary.com). Damn! In regard to sobriety, I tend to think of mercy as something we have to find and have for ourselves. It is difficult because if we did not feel horrible about something we have done as a result of partaking in our addictions, we would not be here, looking for a way to give up those addictions. Even if our motivation is only from a health perspective, what we have done to cause the decline in our health is worthy of needing atonement for our actions. If you are anything like me, you are much harder on yourself than you are on any other person. This makes the idea of having mercy for ourselves more difficult because we most likely feel we are unworthy of it.

I read a lot of posts, tweets, and blogs from people who are struggling to stay on a path of sobriety, and there seems to be one common theme running throughout all of them. The theme is the idea of weakness and the need for help. Whether this is true or not, if we believe we are weak, then we are certain to act in such a way as to prove ourselves correct. It is not to say we have not all felt weak at some point; it's that as long as we do, we are not kind to ourselves. We are not showing ourselves compassion or forgiveness for the fact that we have become addicted to an addictive substance we were told from birth to partake in because it will make our lives better.

The only difference between us and every other person on the planet who is using the substance or participating in the behavior we want to quit is they have not yet reached their bottom. We have, and now it is time for us to take the necessary steps to climb out from our bottom, regain our self-worth, and begin to live a life without the substance or behavior that landed us here in the first place. We cannot concern ourselves with those who are still using; we can only concern ourselves with our journey.

Here is the caveat. Once we have reached our bottom or our non-negotiable point of no return, we have one very big, very important, and very difficult job to do before we can effectively make the changes necessary to heal. We have to show ourselves mercy by showing compassion, offering forgiveness, and loving ourselves, regardless of what we have done in the past. In the movie *28 Days* with Sandra Bullock, one of the patients in rehab says to another patient, "Those are just things you have done. They are not who you are." Our past actions do not define us, but they certainly help guide us when the time comes to find out who and what we want to be in the future.

If you are still struggling to find your path toward sobriety, please do not call yourself weak, do not say you are stupid, do not say you are incapable of quitting; instead, have mercy by showing compassion and forgiveness as you would to your best friend if they were struggling in the same way you are struggling. Love yourself, be kind to yourself, and start telling yourself you are smart, you are strong, you are capable of quitting, and then begin acting in such a way to prove yourself correct.

Have mercy.

Sober - Day 88

The ABCs of Sobriety

When thinking of the word of the day, there was really only one possible option that came to mind, and that word was attached to a piece of writing I read at the beginning of my sober journey. In trying to ensure I am not overstepping legalities with other publications, I reached out to the business and asked if it was okay to write about their book in my blog. I heard back from them, and they said it was fine as long as I credited Annie Grace.

N is for Naked (as in This Naked Mind by Annie Grace)

Definition: adjective; bare, stripped, or destitute; or, without the customary covering or protection (dictionary.com). This feels a little like cheating because I will not be writing as much from my own thoughts, ideas, and beliefs today. I am going to write about someone else's thoughts, ideas, and beliefs, which, to be honest, is pretty much what we do anyway. Most of the time, we develop "[our] own ideas of other people's ideas," as stated by Bo Burnam in his standup special, *Happy*. Nevertheless, Annie Grace's book was the catalyst to why I believe I am enjoying easy sobriety as opposed to hard sobriety, as you have undoubtedly heard me say many times throughout this blog.

Why did This Naked Mind resonate with me?

It was a simple idea, really, and it was an idea I had been working on with my therapist. My therapist and I were exploring the idea of core beliefs and how they affect our relationship to many things, including alcohol. In the introduction, Annie states this as succinctly as possible when she says she is offering, "A perspective that

WILL EMPOWER AND DELIGHT YOU, ALLOWING YOU TO FOREVER CHANGE YOUR RELATIONSHIP WITH ALCOHOL." THAT IS EXACTLY WHAT HER BOOK DID FOR ME; IT CHANGED HOW I LOOKED AT, FELT, BELIEVED, AND SAW ALCOHOL. LET ME ASSURE YOU; I NO LONGER HOLD A KIND NOTION OF ALCOHOL.

It began with her quote, "Alcohol is the only drug you have to make an excuse not to do." This actually angered me to the point I physically felt angst in my heart. I thought to myself, *how can that be possible? How can something as damaging as alcohol be so widely accepted and encouraged that if a person chooses not to do it, they have to feel uncomfortable or make excuses why they are not doing it?* The absurdity in this idea alone should be enough to cause anyone who hears it to voluntarily clear out their liquor cabinets and vow to never support a system of societal peer pressure like the one of alcohol.

The Media Perpetuates the Peer Pressure

While watching a hit television series the other day, I noticed something that blew me away and caused me to take a serious pause while reflecting on the extreme nature of the issue. In the show's rating, they used two words relating to sexuality, just to make sure we don't subject ourselves to that heinous content. They clearly state smoking, which we have known for decades, is truly bad for us. But look at "substances." Why do they use a word so subjective and vague? Other than marijuana (which is becoming widely accepted because of its growing legality), the only "substance" regularly seen in this television show (so far, I'm only on season one) is alcohol. It baffles me that those who make the ratings and parental discretions do not believe alcohol, one of the most addictive and damaging substances we know of, is not worthy of a mention by name.

Are You Angry Yet?

You should be. Everywhere we go, everything we do, every movie we watch, and every book we read has some implicit or explicit mention of alcohol and its "positive" effects on our lives. I could go on and on about how Annie Grace's book *This Naked Mind* outlines all that is wrong with the system of alcohol in our society. In an effort to refrain from writing an unreasonably long blog post, I will end with one of my first experiences after quitting alcohol further substantiating Annie's sentiment about alcohol and its overwhelming social acceptance.

At the beginning of my blog writing, I spent a lot of time writing about my "firsts" without alcohol, so you may have heard this already. Every Tuesday night for the past two years, I have been going to the bowling alley to participate in my bowling league. Now, this is a group of about two hundred people who drink heavily and have no qualms bragging about it. I was one of those people. Needless to say, I was a little apprehensive about going on that first Tuesday after quitting drinking. I walked into the bar to order something non-alcoholic, and, of course, the bartender knew me by name and immediately said hi while simultaneously reaching for the tap containing my favorite beer. I stopped her and told her I was not drinking, to which she replied, "What's the matter? Are you not feeling well?" I said, "No, I quit drinking." To which she and two other servers who knew me responded in unison with, "Oh, don't be a quitter." My jaw fell to the counter. I said something I can't remember, grabbed my O'Doul's, and walked out of the bar without saying another word.

Read the book. I promise you will at least begin to look at alcohol differently, which I believe is the most important asset to the success of our sobriety.

Thank you, Annie Grace, for your wonderful take on sobriety through *This Naked Mind*.

Sober - Day 89

The ABCs of Sobriety

One thing I have learned over the past eighty-nine days is I have caused myself to miss out on an enormous amount of opportunities throughout my life due to my addictions. I definitely cannot say I did not have chances along the way to better my life, to explore new passions, to experience new things, or to meet new people. We all do, probably every single day. We have moments that come up and give us the chance to make a choice; we either go for it, or we do not. Unfortunately, I spent most of my life not going for it. Not anymore.

O is for Opportunity

Definition: noun; an occasion or situation that makes it possible to do something that you want to or have to do (dictionary.com). I was not expecting this blog to go in this direction, but I am suddenly overwhelmed with the idea of choice. Opportunity is certainly the word of the day, but the choice we make is ultimately what gives it its power. Otherwise, it is just another unremarkable event that occurs, and we either experience it, or we do not. An opportunity presents us with a choice to do something we want or have to do. In regard to sobriety, I would have to suggest the opportunity is to do something we have to do.

How do we know when an opportunity presents itself?

I would have to say this is the most difficult aspect to discern. First, we have to be open to the idea it is possible to have a moment or moments aligning for us and placing us in a mental state to enact change. This goes back to the deserving part of sobriety. We have to believe we deserve it and we are worthy of it in order to see it occur. I believe most often, the opportunities we have missed or allowed to pass us by are simply a result of our mind's inability to see them take shape. We can only truly see what we believe to be true.

Second, once we see an opportunity present itself, we have to recognize it for what it is: an opportunity to do something we have to do. For addicts, this means to walk away from the thing stripping us down and leaving us hanging by a thread. This is by no means easy for anyone, but we are surrounded every day by people who have not only recognized the opportunity to make a change but who have taken the opportunity and effectively used it to open new doors, paths, and a potential they never knew possible. Look for those people and reach out to them. Open yourself up to meeting them. I am proud to say I am one of those people. It took me a while because I fought it for as long as I possibly could. Eventually, however, the fighting wore me down, and I could no longer ignore the fact opportunity was staring me in the face every single day of my life. You know what opportunity is called? Today.

Today is our opportunity

Every day we wake up is a new day that is offered to us as an opportunity to make the changes necessary to live the life we have always wanted to live. We have had a feeling stirring in our gut for as long as we can remember. You know the feeling I am referring to; it's the feeling that tells us deep down in our soul we are meant for something bigger. I know it is hard to accept the feeling as truth. I know it because I remember how detached I felt from the feeling when I first felt it. It felt so vastly far away from me. Even if I wanted to believe it, it was too far away to ever reach. I was certain no matter how fast I ran, how hard I tried, and no matter what I did, the idea of a better version of me would just keep drifting away like a life raft blowing downstream, just out of reach.

MAKE THE CHOICE TO ACCEPT THE OPPORTUNITY

The difference, I am not afraid to say, is choice. If you don't make the choice to accept the challenge of the opportunity laid before you, then the life raft will just continue to blow out of your reach. Stop struggling to reach it. Choose to reach it. It is in your right, power, and will to make the choice to change your life and subsequently the lives of everyone around you. Your strength becomes someone else's strength, and so on. Opportunity is a perpetual wheel of positive and life-changing potential, and it starts with you.

Your opportunity for change is today. Accept it.

SOBER - DAY 90

THE ABCS OF SOBRIETY

If you have been following me at all, you do not even have to guess what the word of the day is for today's blog. I have been fascinated by it, talking about it, trying to understand it better, and I've been pretty much obsessed with it. How could I not? It is the single most important aspect of not only sobriety but of every single thing we do in our daily lives. I love talking about it, learning about it, hearing about it, and living while constantly considering its power. It is the one true answer to every question and problem we encounter throughout our lives.

P IS FOR PERSPECTIVE

Definition: noun; a particular attitude toward or way of regarding something; a point of view (dictionary.com). Just for fun, I decided to look up the phrase "point of view" as well: an opinion, attitude, or judgment. At this point, my therapist just laughs when I bring up how engrossed I am with this concept. She doesn't laugh at me; she laughs because we talked about it for a year and a half before it finally sank in. Now it has, and it's all I want to talk about it. I said in the first paragraph it is the answer to all problems, which might be a little lofty, but I don't believe it is by much.

How does perspective relate to alcohol?

I have talked about this a lot, but I don't believe it can ever be heard too often, especially for those of us in our early stages of sobriety. Look again at the definition: a particular attitude toward something. Ask yourself right now, what is your relationship with alcohol? If you answer with any form of positive feelings toward the substance, then you are holding on to something forever making abstaining difficult. If you miss it, then you mourn its absence, and therefore, set yourself up for failure. Here is the tricky part: I don't believe you can hate it, either. How many things in our lives have we hated and continued to do, consume, or allow in our lives? If we give a lot of energy and time to something, it will continue to manifest itself in our lives every day.

Don't hate alcohol, understand it

By understanding what alcohol is and how it affects our lives, bodies, and relationships, we take power away from it. If we change our attitude toward it, then our perception changes about its role in our lives. How can we hold a positive feeling toward something literally killing our loved ones and us every day? We can't if we see it for what it is. If we continue to hold on to the opinion shoved down our throats from childhood that alcohol is good, it helps us calm down, it makes us more fun; it makes us funnier, it makes us more social, it is something we deserve, then we will continue to view it as a positive influence in our lives. Our perception of alcohol gives it power, or it takes it away.

Understanding alcohol is literally poison is one thing, but understanding it actually does none of the things listed above is another. Alcohol does, in fact, lower our inhibitions and limits our defense mechanisms, which allow us to feel more "brave." It does numb our physical and emotional feelings, making us feel stronger, and it certainly encourages us to do things we may never do sober. It does create a sense of security, making us feel more "ourselves." Let's honestly look at what all those things really mean.

Rather than talk about the science behind how alcohol is a false security blanket, I'll explain what I have witnessed since I quit drinking that allows me to understand how none of the "benefits" stated above are actually true. The more I socialize sober with people who are drinking, the more I realize how much of what I always thought about alcohol is truly a fallacy. The people I used to think were hysterical, are really not very funny. The idea I could not dance without drinking was self-imposed; the truth is, I actually dance better sober than I ever did drunk because I have all my faculties in order. The idea I was able to socialize better was complete nonsense because now I am able to recall information on the fly. I am able to form coherent thoughts and actually make sense. I am able to hold a truly intellectual conversation about subjects other than booze, food, personal conquests, and partying.

The worst of the alcohol lies is the idea alcohol calms us down. Yes, it does numb our nervous system and shuts down our thought processes, but that is only temporary. The moment it wears off, we are hungover, feel like shit, and have less confidence about handling life stresses than we did before we started drinking. The only option we have at this point is to drink more to dull the pain we feel instigated from the previous night's drinking and begin the whole cycle over again. Oh, and we never actually dealt with or solved the catalyst for the stress causing us to drink in the first place.

Alcohol Has Been Gaslighting Us and We Didn't Even Know It

Of course, until we change our perception of our relationship with alcohol, our trusty little "friend" will continue to beat us up every day. It will tear us down and cause us to lose ourselves, our friends, and our family. It will ensure we always rely on it because that is how it receives its power. It makes us feel we need it when, in fact, what we really need is to see the lies it and society have been telling us since we were born.

Alcohol is not our friend, but remember, do not see it as the enemy, either because we fight with our enemies. See it for what it is; it is then you will understand you no longer need to fight with it; you are above it, and so begins the first steps toward "easy sobriety."

Sober - Day 91

The ABCs of Sobriety

It's another Sober Friday, and the only thing better than a Sober Friday is a Sober Saturday when I wake up and feel refreshed and ready to tackle all my goals, intentions, and projects. Sober mornings just never get old. Occasionally, I wake up a little dehydrated from not drinking enough water, and I feel a little fogginess in my head. I have a momentary panic attack, and then I remember it's not because I drank too much. I continue about my day with still more energy than I ever did on my best hangover days. You just can't beat living a life filled with energy, aspirations, dreams, intentions, and productivity.

Q IS FOR QUALITY

Definition: noun; the standard of something as measured against other things of a similar kind; the degree of excellence of something (dictionary.com). This can be taken in several different ways and in several different contexts, but I believe the most important standard the alcoholic and addict must measure something against is their own past. I teach my son to never compare himself to others in regard to his happiness, and I think it applies here, too. You could look at friends or family who have become sober and compare and contrast their experience with yours, but I think the best comparison you can ever make is to compare your life when you were drinking with where you are now (or want to be). I say want to be because some of you may not be where you want to be yet, and, therefore, do not have the alternative comparison. If this is the case, then imagine what you want your life to look like after quitting alcohol or other addictions and concentrate on the quality of your life until you achieve it.

THE "QUALITY" OF THE ADDICTED LIFE

Since the definition refers to measuring two things, I figure it makes sense to look at life while using first and see how it makes us feel. I will talk about my life since I am an expert in that area and have a little insight to offer. But it is all relative, isn't it? My life didn't look that bad, but I was in bad shape physically, mentally, and emotionally. I had three addictions, and probably more, if I am honest, and they were simply destroying my ability to live a life of "quality." The nicotine was controlling too much of my thoughts because, as I mentioned before, I was trying not to do it on the sly, and that meant I had to constantly be aware of when and how I would get my next fix. It felt like a full-time job, and when I found myself in times where I couldn't use it, I panicked and felt terribly anxious.

Alcohol was literally controlling my every move. I was waking up in the morning with only the thought of when I was going to be able to drink. I did not, mostly, drink at inappropriate times, but I absolutely could not wait until I was able to allow myself to consume alcohol. This meant the rearranging of my day and responsibilities at times to ensure I could drink earlier and as much as I wanted. I woke up thinking about drinking, I went through my day thinking about drinking, I talked about drinking, I bragged about drinking, and I pretty much lived to drink. It was very important to me and my identity. One evening at bowling, after quitting, my partner made fun of me for not drinking anymore because only a couple of weeks prior, I made this comment, "I don't trust people who don't drink." What the fuck? Just typing those words gives me chills. Who holds such an opinion?

My other addiction was more behaviorally related. It was another "time suck," as I like to call it, it just took up entirely too much of my time and kept me from doing all the things I wanted to do. It was something holding me down as much as the substances, but it was harder to let go of because it did not carry the same negative physical qualities as alcohol and nicotine. I had to find other ways to see it, too, was detracting from the quality of my life, and I needed to let it go as well. It doesn't really matter what it is; if you see something as a negative in your life, then you must consider letting it go. I needed to let it go, too, and I did.

The Quality of the Sober Life

Sobriety has brought with it a quality of life I never knew possible. I know I have said this time and time again throughout my blog, but it is the most truthful statement I know. What is the difference in my life now? I no longer spend any amount of time thinking about negative ways to destroy my body, mind, and life. I no longer waste my time doing things that do not benefit me, my family, or my future. I am in constant motion toward healing and progress in all areas of my life. I now set goals and achieve them. I set intentions and watch them occur. I live a life of positivity, abundance, joy, gratitude, and kindness. I am living the quality of life I never knew I wanted because I never knew I could achieve it. Sobriety is the biggest gift I have ever given myself, and I will spend the rest of my life showing gratitude for that gift.

As a side note, and because of the predicament we, as a society, find ourselves in due to the pandemic outbreak, I would be remiss not to mention how the quality of life during this quarantine would have been different had I still been using. I honestly cannot even imagine what a train wreck I would have been if I had not made the decision to quit all my addictions before this occurred. I would have been drinking too much every day. I would have been full of anxiety, trying to use nicotine while trying to keep it from L. I would have felt like shit every day, and I would have probably gained twenty pounds just from boredom. Worst of all, I would not have taken advantage of the time to better myself as a person.

Alternatively, I have exercised every day and finally established working out as part of my lifestyle again. I have read several books, including Quitlit and novels. I have written a blog every day and I am going to turn my blogs into a book. I have almost finished a full-length novel. I have taken on writing work as an editor, a ghostwriter, and I have been accepted to write articles for an online writing firm. My wife and I have gotten along magnificently. She quit drinking, too, and I have spent way more time with my son doing things he enjoys as well as things we enjoy as a family. While I hate the negativity occurring in the world due to this unfortunate virus outbreak, I have not let it bring my family or me down, and we have made the most out of a bad situation.

If you are reading this, you are most likely not happy with at least one aspect or quality of your life. I am here to personally tell you life without addiction equals the highest quality of life you can imagine. Take control of your life and live the life of your dreams.

Sober - Day 92

The ABCs of Sobriety

Throughout my short time in sobriety, I have witnessed and heard a lot of talk about the word of the day. I believe it is actually somewhat controversial in the sober community, which, of course, is right up my alley. I can have an open mind and understand the origin of the word in the context of sobriety. I can even say there is some merit to it, but as I continue to move forward in my sobriety and witness people struggle, I think it is time to do away with this word in the sober community. I say this because I think it carries only negativity. From the addict's vantage point, the last thing an addict needs is more negativity.

R is for Relapse

Definition: verb; a deterioration of someone's state of health after a temporary improvement (dictionary.com). The problem I have with this word is not so much whether or not it relates accurately to the idea of sobriety, but whether or not it is helpful in the idea of sobriety. From a technical standpoint, yes, a relapse is a deterioration because a person now has alcohol in their system after a period of abstinence from the poisonous chemical. But does the action honestly deserve the negative stigma that follows it in some of the sober communities I have recently witnessed? I don't believe it does.

How does the sober community view a relapse?

Unfortunately, the traditional sober community places a lot of emphasis on days of sobriety, which makes sense based on the way their program is designed, "one day at a time." I don't have any problem with this at all. And, if I am honest, I am contradicting myself a little based on the title of my blogs, Sober - Day (blank). I just like the way it sounded; it wasn't necessarily meant to be a counter. Anyway, the problem I do have with the importance placed on how many days a person has sober is over time, it may become somewhat of an identity. What happens when a person who relates wholly to a particular identity suddenly loses their identity because they simply make a mistake? People making "mistakes" is generally considered a normal fact of life and even celebrated as a learning or teaching moment in every other aspect of the human condition. Why, then, do addicts, the people who actually need the most forgiveness, connection, and understanding, not receive the same consideration in sobriety?

It seems, in the sober community, the word "relapse" is synonymous with failure. I believe failure is the worst emotion an addict can feel when actively taking positive steps toward healing and a better life. If we make a mistake in any other avenue of our lives, we are only considered a failure if we do not learn something from the mistake. If we do learn something and then apply what we have learned toward our next attempt, we are considered a success, or at the very least, on the road to success. We are certainly not considered a failure for making a mistake. What would happen if we applied this same concept to the idea of sobriety?

Relapse is simply a teaching moment

Obviously, having a drink after abstaining from alcohol for a period of time is not going to feel good or help build confidence. But, neither does falling off a horse. What is the old saying, "Get back on the horse"? That saying, interestingly enough, is really the true determining factor of whether or not a person has failed in their sobriety. If we get back up, and no matter how reluctantly we make an effort to swing our leg back over the horse and try again, we have *not* failed. It is the action of giving up wholly that places a person back where they started. It is at that point the word "failure" becomes relevant.

As long as we continue to learn, try, and seek help and understanding for our addiction, we are not failing. We are simply taking active steps to find our own personal path to sobriety. Let me assure you—there is no single set path to sobriety. I do believe, however, there are easier paths than others, and that belief has somehow solidified itself in my mind as a personal quest to find and unveil. It is the evasive and elusive path to what I like to call "easy sobriety."

Take it easy on yourself and others. Be kind and forgive each other for being human. We are fallible, and the sooner we accept our fallibility, the sooner we can take the necessary steps down the unknown path secretly lying before us. With any luck, we will inevitably find the right fork in the road allowing us to feel we have finally found our emotional home. I say inevitable because it is just a matter of time.

As long as we keep trying, we are *not* failing.

SOBER - DAY 93

THE ABCS OF SOBRIETY

There are so many separate things attached to the word of the day I believe someone could write an entire book on it if one were so inclined. If you are like me, you have walked through life pretty unaware of what you were capable of and too afraid to really ever take the risk to find out. When things did go well, you experienced the "imposter syndrome" and never really trusted the good fortune was meant for you because you did nothing to deserve it. Unfortunately, the inability to see, accept, and trust in today's word is really one of the most poignant facets of sobriety and, subsequently, recovery.

S is for Self

Definition: noun; a person's essential being that distinguishes them from others, especially considered as the object of introspection or reflective action (dictionary.com). Oh my, what a wonderful definition. I especially love the idea of the object of introspection and reflective action. How perfectly does it fit into the ABCs of Sobriety and play a role in recovery? I can't think of a better word, actually.

Self-doubt

This is where most of us started this whole debacle of spiraling out of control until hitting a bottom of some sort. I can truthfully say while going through the first forty-eight years of my life I did not believe in myself because I had no idea what I was made of. I don't know how some people seem to be born with a strong sense of self, and others seem to have figuratively missed the class, but it is clear there are two defining types of people in the world. There are people with a strong sense of self, and then there are the rest of us.

The obvious problem with self-doubt is if we hold an opinion of self-doubt in our minds and we continue to tell ourselves we don't believe in ourselves, then our minds will inevitably agree and ensure it to be true. That is all the time I am going to spend on the negative aspect of self.

Self-worth

When talking about self, there are so many avenues we could traverse down, but I think for the sake of sobriety, I will focus on a couple I believe to be essential in recovery and, ultimately, sobriety. Self-worth was the tallest and most challenging hurdle I had to face while finding my true self. I just couldn't see it. I could not believe I had anything to offer. I could not see that I was strong, determined, and just as capable of success as anyone else. I did not believe I deserved to be happy.

Self-worth. I do not fully understand how quitting drinking affected my self-worth so dramatically, but it did. I think it was simply a way of showing myself I was strong, I could choose to make things happen, I had determination, and I could resolve to do anything I wanted. The difference between not understanding your worth and knowing it can be illustrated by the following. Ask yourself these questions and fill in the blanks, "Do I deserve to be _____? Do I deserve to have _____? Do I deserve to feel _____?" If you hesitate on any of those questions, then you are probably struggling with some aspect of your self-worth, and that's okay. But, you *have* to change your perception in regard to your self-worth before you can truly make the changes that directly correlate to your recovery and sobriety.

Alcohol, nicotine, destructive behaviors, and any other addictions have one job; they keep you from finding your true self. They keep you in a state of depression and feeling worthless so you cannot garner the strength necessary to overcome your weaknesses. In order to feel a higher level of self-worth, you must take the power and control back.

SELF-CONFIDENCE

Once you have begun to see, trust, and understand your increasing level of self-worth, you then begin to feel your self-confidence grow, and this is fucking remarkable. How many times have you seen something you wanted or something you wanted to do but then told yourself, "I cannot have or do that"? Why would we tell ourselves this? We do it because it is easier to deal with the idea we don't have the capacity for something rather than the idea we tried to obtain it and failed. It's a self-preservation technique effectively keeping us from finding our true selves and happiness.

Self-confidence is the emotion propelling us past any thought of cannot and into a perpetual thought of can. We can do anything we want if we believe it to be true. That is self-confidence. Let me show you what I mean. I have recently proclaimed something I believe in my heart and soul to be true. I believe it so strongly I am already taking steps to prepare for what my life is going to feel and be like based on the changes resulting from this proclamation. Ready?

I am a full-time professional writer.

Hold my non-alcoholic beer and watch this.

Sober - Day 94

The ABCs of Sobriety

As I continue to envelop my life with the sober community, I keep seeing the same underlying themes come up. Some of those themes I have already written about here. It is the recurring themes keeping me invested in writing about my experiences, reading about others' experiences, and talking to people to try and better understand their experiences. I want to understand why these recurring themes keep coming up, time and time again. I believe there are a couple of culprits, but I think it is the less obvious ones really tripping us up on our road to recovery and sobriety. Today's word is one of those culprits, and it is one that is really not that easy to change; until it is.

T IS FOR THOUGHTS

Definition: noun; an idea or opinion produced by thinking or occurring suddenly in the mind (dictionary.com). I have read the average person has up to 6,200 thoughts every single day (newshub.com). That is a lot of thinking, especially for those of us who don't really think we think as much as we think. Anyway, there are bound to be some negative thoughts creeping up in all that mess throughout the day, so how do we keep our minds thinking positively all the time? I imagine this is the question of the millennium. I don't know if it is a matter of not thinking negatively as much as it is a matter of focusing on the positive more often than the negative.

I recently read and watched *The Secret* again, and they spent a lot of time talking about how thoughts become things. I am currently practicing this technique in my own life, and what I have learned is it is very difficult for a person suffering from addiction to hold thoughts that differ greatly from what they are experiencing at a given moment. Let's look at the definition again: an opinion produced by thinking. The opinion, in this case, is what we believe about ourselves. If we hold a negative opinion of ourselves, we will believe it and make it true. If we hold a positive opinion about ourselves, we will believe it and make it true, also.

HOW DO WE EFFECTIVELY AFFECT OUR THOUGHT PATTERNS?

I follow a lot of social media these days as I search for truths and information about addiction, sobriety, and recovery. Today I saw two posts in a matter of minutes inspiring me to write about thoughts this morning. The first was a post on a sober page that said, "Why me? Why can't I be done with this already? Why am I so weak?" There are three reaffirming statements in that one sentence telling a person what their opinion of themselves is: a victim, who is impatient and weak. How can our minds ever think about ourselves positively with those thoughts swimming around in a consistent swirl of negativity? It can't.

Can we monitor every negative thought we have?

No, of course not. But we can focus on the positive and post about it instead, right? Think about how much energy went into the above post. They had to first have the thought, then think about the thought enough times to form a structured idea. Then, they had to pull out their phone or computer with the intent of writing about the thought, and then type the thought into a couple of sentences which they probably had to edit a few times to get right. That is a lot of focus and energy on negative thoughts. How differently might the person's day have gone had they performed all of the same actions and thinking that led instead to a different post? "I am strong. I am on the right path. I believe in me." Those are the kinds of thoughts that affect change.

The other post I saw today came in the form of a message. I had asked someone in my Facebook group if they were feeling strong. Their response was, "Yes, surprisingly." To which I responded, "Start there; it is not surprising because you are a badass, and you can do anything you want." I know it is hard to change our thoughts—believe me, I am still working on all of this myself. But it is like anything else we want to become better at; it takes practice. First, just try and recognize negative thoughts. Once you notice one, try and stop yourself for a moment and ask yourself how you could reframe the thought to inject some positivity into your thinking. Even if you don't really believe it yet, just reframe the thought and say it. I promise it will get easier, and more importantly, you will begin to believe it.

Thoughts are Everything

I know it sounds a bit cheesy and somewhat superlative, but what if it is true? I can honestly and emphatically say in my relatively short time working through changing my mindset, perception, and thinking, I have personally seen this to be true. I am learning how to change my mood simply by changing the thoughts in my head. This is how I change a negative mood into a positive one. First, I literally say thank you for as many things as I can come up with in a short amount of time. Then, I go through my list of intentions for how I want to live my life. I say them as if I am doing or already have done them like this: I am a professional writer. I have written books on the *New York Times* Bestsellers List. I am a great husband and father, etc. I do those two things until I begin to smile, and I inevitably begin to smile every single time. It takes a little practice, but it works.

Manipulate your thoughts until your thoughts manipulate your world.

Sober - Day 95

The ABCs of Sobriety

I have used this quote by Johan Hari before because I believe it to be a highly unique (and no, that is not the word for U) take on the perception of addiction: "The opposite of addiction is not sobriety; the opposite of addiction is connection." We forget so easily the things that brought some of us to our addiction and spend more time focusing on what is wrong with us. If the human condition is prone to suffering alone, then it makes sense in a self-isolating world we could easily succumb to the lies perpetuated by the promises society and alcohol have made to us. Once we use an addiction to "heal" our loneliness, our loneliness grows deeper until we lose all semblance of the social being we once were.

U IS FOR UNITY

Definition: noun; the state of being united or joined as a whole (dictionary.com). For our purposes here, the unity I am speaking of is the unity created by a sober community. I have been amazed by the number of resources available to a person seeking a community to help with their sobriety. I immediately began to seek a community through social media when I first quit in the hopes of meeting like-minded people, hearing their stories, and ultimately building up an arsenal of people I could rely on if times grew too difficult or if I just needed someone to lean on. I have certainly found my community.

I thought for today's blog, and in honor of today's word, unity, I would talk about some of the resources I have found while on my sober journey. Unfortunately, I was unable to find a community of real-life people in my circle of friends. I imagine this is not too uncommon because we tend to migrate toward people who hold similar beliefs and values to our own. Obviously, for addicts, this creates a conundrum for our recovery and eventual sobriety unless we find other ways to create a community of support. Make no mistake—we must find a community of support.

LITERATURE

This may not be what you were expecting when thinking of community, but there is a method to my madness. The very first book I picked up, and you have heard this before, was *This Naked Mind* by Annie Grace. It was the book that changed the way I saw alcohol and it provided me the new lens through which to approach all of my addictions. What I quickly learned while and after reading the book was there were an enormous amount of people who have read the book, too. They were all searching for others who have read the book so they could talk about their experiences and share time with like-minded people. In fact, the first day I quit and started reading Annie Grace's book, I found she also has an online community resource. It has been very beneficial to me and countless others. It is the This Naked Mind community. Check it out. She also holds classes, seminars and does videos to help anyone still struggling. This is an amazing resource.

The second piece of literature I read was We Are the Luckiest by Laura McKowen. You might remember me talking about how this book made me breakdown and cry in the introduction. Her words touched me because, through her experience, I was able to see my future, and it is a future I have always dreamed I wanted but never thought I was capable of achieving. Now, I am achieving my dreams, and I will forever be thankful to her for her part in my recovery and sobriety. She, too, offers seminars, online meetings, and other resources for people still struggling with sobriety.

ONLINE RESOURCES

This is an avenue where a person can certainly get lost because there are literally thousands of resources online for people searching for unity through a sober community. I would suggest taking your time and looking through all that is available out there. In my experience, there are a lot of beliefs and opinions for the "right" way to approach recovery and sobriety, and some of them are downright aggressive. I am certain there is something out there for everyone, so be patient and try and find the "thing" that works best for you.

I found a couple of helpful groups on Facebook I will not link to because I feel it is something you need to search for and feel out for yourself. I also found Twitter, surprisingly, held a lot of support in the way of a community through which a person could find unity. Instagram is another good platform through which to find sober communities. The tags

I have found the most useful on Twitter and Instagram are #sober #soberlife #sobriety #alcoholfree, and #recovery, though there are many more.

I will go ahead and shamelessly plug the work I have been doing, too, because I have received a lot of positive feedback, and it seems people are relating to what I am trying to put out there. I do the best I can to be available and to hold meetings a couple of times a week; even when nobody shows, I am still there. It is a way of being of service, something I did very little while using. I would appreciate any and all of your support in spreading the word of my work thus far. You are all appreciated. Here are my links, once again:

https://linktr.ee/xstopwriting

There really are an enormous amount of resources out there for anyone wishing to find unity through a sober community. Take the time to find what works for you and use it as a way to keep yourself accountable for the goals you are setting for yourself in recovery and sobriety. Living a sober life is the best decision I have ever made, and I am sure it will be for you as well, especially if you can find a supportive community to help you find the success you deserve.

SOBER - DAY 96

THE ABCS OF SOBRIETY

There is a saying by Walter Benjamin, "History is written by the victor." If this is true, then whoever wins in a battle has the power to write what history took place leading up to the present. This is quite poignant in the battle over addiction because one of the most common sentiments I hear is how people regret, feel bad about, hate, and can't forget the wrongs they have done in their past, which makes up their own personal history. Today's word, if taken literally, tells us that is no longer the case.

V IS FOR VICTORY

Definition: noun; the act of defeating an enemy or an opponent in a battle, game, or other competition (dictionary.com). Is there a greater enemy than addiction? Well, there might be, but not for the addict, of course. While we can all agree fighting addiction is not a game or even something we would consider a competition, it is certainly a battle, and for most of us, one of the biggest battles we will ever face. The good news? Emerging victorious in this battle allows us to rewrite our own personal history because we, my friend, are the victor.

IT'S TIME TO LET GO OF OUR PAST

Yes, we all have them, and if you are an addict, you most likely have a very colorful one. We could all talk for hours about all the stupid shit we have done while using; we have a lot from which to draw. One of the things I am desperately trying to do for myself and in my Facebook group is to focus more on the positive aspects of sobriety. Let's spend our energy talking about what we want, what we enjoy about sobriety, what we want for our future, and how we can support each other in all the positive existing in sobriety because there is a lot.

While attending some online sober meetings, I realized pretty quickly the majority of the time was spent listening to someone's struggles and disparaging stories about all the bad things they have done. Interestingly enough, we all laugh at these stories because they are familiar, and we know we have been in those same shoes, but is this where we want our focus, especially in the early stages of sobriety? I don't believe that is the best use of our energy. What I noticed from those meetings was at the end of a person's share, there was always a snippet of positivity I found myself wanting to cheer for, reach out and (virtually) hug the person, and tell them congratulations. Isn't this where we should want to spend our energy?

Focus on Today and the Future, but Mostly Today

I say mostly today because, obviously, the future is unwritten, and we never know what is going to happen, but we can shape the future. How do we do this? It all comes down to our decisions and behaviors. For addicts, I am speaking directly to our decisions and behaviors around our addictions. Laura McKowen tells a story in her book, *We Are the Luckiest* about a time in a yoga teaching class. A student told the instructor they didn't think they could quit drinking. The yoga instructor simply said, "Of course you can; are you drinking now?" The student replied no, and the teacher continued to ask the same question, "How about now?" Until the idea set in for the whole class, and they all smiled from understanding. The point is, the "now" the instructor was asking about is the present. If you are not drinking right now, it is because you are choosing not to drink at this moment. Whether your choice to not drink is because you are in a yoga class, at work, driving, with your children, or in a venue that does not allow alcohol, you are making that choice not to drink. The reason may be because drinking in those circumstances is unsafe, not socially accepted, unhealthy, or just plain stupid. But, you are making the choice nonetheless, and you can make the choice in every moment of every day for the rest of your life. When you do this, you are victorious.

Rewrite Your History

Starting today, with every positive decision you make and every drink you do not drink, you begin a new story of your life. The new story will be much more fulfilling, exciting, gratifying, and affirming than any story you can dredge up from your past. Your present will invigorate your resolve to maintain sobriety because you will feel confidence grow inside of you. You will begin to get to know your true self. You will see you are actually a pretty fucking cool person without alcohol. You will rewrite your past by living well in the present and creating a new storyline anyone would be proud and happy to live and share in the future.

Victory: the act of defeating an enemy. I am going to do something a little different to end this blog than I have in the past. There is a song by Disturbed that has been inspiring me when looking at defeating addiction or just bad energy. You may not care for metal music, but the sentiment is pretty awesome. It's called "Conflict." Check it out.

https://www.youtube.com/watch?v=PUJT9unnDok

If it doesn't work for you, I understand. It is not for everyone. Just go out and remember the one essential question, "Are you drinking now? No? How about now?"

Sober - Day 97

The ABCs of Sobriety

I fell in love with the idea for today's word the moment I woke up and remembered what letter I was on for today's ABCs of Sobriety blog entry. It really embodies the reasoning behind most of our choices to find a path toward sobriety, but it also means a very different thing in the majority of its normal colloquial usage. In order to truly understand it from the lens I would like to speak through today, you will have to have been in a place in your life, at some point, where you felt as though you and your life held very little value. It is from that place you can really see and feel the difference between the addict's view and the colloquial view of the word.

W is for Wealth

Definition: noun; a great quantity or store of money, valuable possessions, property, or other riches (dictionary.com). If you think I am about to write about the first three of those items, you probably don't want to continue. I believe I speak for most of my sober colleagues who have or are traversing their sobriety path, the idea of money, property, or possessions was the last thing on our minds when making the elusive decision to finally take the step onto our sober paths. It's the "other riches" I would like to speak to today.

What is wealth, if not money?

While we can all agree money is very important to our lives as we negotiate the acceptable norms of living in a civilized society, it is certainly not the most important aspect of wealth. However, when looking around the world today, it is safe to say the idea of wealth being anything other than money is slowly losing its value. Just look at the sheer number of choices for every single thing we want or need to buy. From an economic standpoint, the ridiculous number of choices we now have comes from the demand placed on the market by our consumer-based lifestyles. Do the hundreds of different options for cell phones increase the quality of our lives? No, but people are certainly willing to pay an enormous amount of money for something that does very little different from its competitors. Money equals wealth and, therefore, better potential for happiness. Right? I spend an enormous amount of my parenting time trying to help my son see this is wrong.

For the addict, whose life has consisted of uncertainty, struggle, loss, pain, and a complete lack of confidence, wealth has a much different meaning. We stopped worrying about money, possessions, and property long ago and instead spent our time worrying more about survival. I don't know how many times I thought about the potential of letting go of my addictions and what it would mean for my overall quality of life. Not once did the idea of money ever encroach on any of those thoughts. My idea of wealth while using was having a semblance of control over my life and actions, doing things I loved to do, loving and being present with my family and friends, accomplishing goals I never thought possible, and even just experiencing a simple sense of peace and calmness in my mind and heart. That would have been my definition of wealth back then, and you know what, that is still my definition of wealth today.

WEALTH IN SOBRIETY IS INTERNAL

I have worked in a career making over six figures. I have had opportunities to experience how the traditional concept of wealth affects a person's life. I get it, understand it, and I even condone the idea of trying to obtain it, as long as it does not require you to veer from your moral compass.

Let me tell you about the greatest amount of wealth I have ever held. It began on January 18, 2020, when I made the decision to quit drinking, stay off nicotine, and refrain from other addictive behaviors negatively affecting my life. Since that day, my personal emotional wealth has grown exponentially in the form of self-worth, confidence, happiness, love, joy, friendship, family, goal achievement, and a myriad of other self-perpetuating actions contributing to my overall growth as a human being. In ninety-seven days, I went from having no goals to establishing and putting into place a course of action that will allow me to enact every single thing I want for my life and the life of my family. I am living a life of abundance because, for the first time in my life, I understand and believe in the true meaning of wealth.

And it has nothing to do with money.

Sober - Day 98

The ABCs of Sobriety

I have had a little bit of a difficult time this morning with today's letter of the day. It is not the easiest word for which to come up with something clever or inspiring. With that said, I decided to go with a variation of the letter in a word that relates to sobriety before I stress myself out getting too far behind in my morning routine. Once I gave myself permission to veer from the exact letter a little bit, I came up with many options I could work with but ultimately landed on a word I believe is directly related to what we all want from sobriety.

X is for eXcel

Definition: verb; to be exceptionally good at or proficient in an activity or subject (dictionary.com). It is not so much I want us to worry about being exceptionally good at sobriety, although that does correlate here, too, it is more about how sobriety allows us to excel in everything else. Think about it. How many things or aspects of your life were you doing exceptionally well while using besides using? We were all way too good at that. As far as everything else, I was not excelling at anything.

Why is it so difficult to excel while using? I think there are a lot of reasons, but the most obvious for me was alcohol simply killed any motivation I had. My biggest motivation, especially at the end, was the motivation to drink. I planned my days around it and went to extreme measures to ensure I had access to it in times where my ability to drink was inhibited. Other than that, I simply went through life perpetually buzzed or drunk, with a headache and always tired. I was tired because I think my body would wake me up at three in the morning wanting more alcohol, and I couldn't get back to sleep. It is hard to believe this could be true, but I don't know how to explain the lack of sleep I was struggling with before I quit. Now I sleep through the night and wake feeling refreshed and ready to go. With all that going on, how could I ever feel motivated to excel at anything? I couldn't.

Where can I excel in life after alcohol?

Anywhere and everywhere!

Take your pick. I have talked about how time was an unexpected benefit of sobriety. It is amazing how much time you gain back in your day when you are not using. I am not trying to over-exaggerate here, but it is extraordinary. The time starts when you wake up feeling good all the way throughout your day and into the evening when you choose to go to bed rather than pass out. How many hours have you spent on a sofa drinking and watching television every day before passing out? For me, it is an excruciating reality to admit, but it is true. The time you gain back in your life affords you the opportunity to begin working on all those things you have been putting off or too afraid to begin.

Once you begin using your time wisely, you will begin to see just how many things you are truly good at doing, let alone exceptional at doing. This does not have to be some grand idea either, like writing a book or graduating college. It could be something as simple and important as excelling at being a parent, a partner, or a friend. I did pretty well at being a parent, but I do not think I was very good at being a partner or friend. I was too consumed with my own failures and lack of self-worth to give any energy to someone else. Looking back, I truly miss the time I threw away there, but I am and will continue to make up for it now.

A PERSONAL EXAMPLE

Here is where I feel I have begun to excel in life since quitting drinking. First, I am a better father and husband; there is no question. I take time to be with my family, and I am more present than I have ever been. I noticed this immediately during the quarantine when I had my son for two weeks, and we spent a lot more quality time together. That is worth any discomfort quitting may have ever caused me. My wife and I spend more quality time together, too; we definitely laugh more, and we rarely miscommunicate anymore because we have the faculties to be articulate. I am more patient at my job and with life and myself. I have set massive goals I am actively taking steps to achieve. I feel good about who I am as a person, and I am proud of what I have accomplished so far as well as what I am accomplishing now. I walk through life with a more positive outlook. I am more capable of finding the good in bad situations. I genuinely care about people. All of these things I had no time for nor the motivation or energy to spend on while using.

One of my favorite changes has been the desire to reach out and help people. I am new to this, but for the first time in my life, I have a very large desire to help people who are struggling, especially with alcohol. I feel I have a lot to offer, and I am in a position in my life to be available to others. I love the connections I am making and the time spent talking about all the positives of quitting addictions. Each person I meet, each story I tell, and each new experience I have reinvigorates my resolve to continue excelling in my life alcohol-free.

Come join me!

Sober - Day 99

The ABCs of Sobriety

Oh my God! I am on day ninety-nine of my 101 days of sobriety blog. I have no idea where the time went; although, I do have a whole lot to show for it. I have already decided, like my thirty-day blog goal, I am not going to stop writing at 101 days either. Hopefully, this makes more of you happy than not. It makes me happy, so I guess that is really all that matters. Nonetheless, I have really enjoyed this process. More than anything, I have enjoyed your comments and support. It has been wonderful knowing something helping me is also helping others. What a blessing.

I have talked at length about today's word of the day for the ABCs of Sobriety. Surprisingly, Y was much more difficult than I was expecting. I thought about a couple of options like you, yield, and yesterday, but none of them struck me as a really good word that correlates with recovery and sobriety. Then, I accidentally happened upon the word I ended up choosing, and it made a lot of sense to me because I believe it is the reason we end up here in the first place. By here, I mean in recovery seeking sobriety.

Y is for Yearn

Definition: verb; to have an intense feeling or longing for something, typically something that one has lost or been separated from (dictionary.com). I almost went with "yesterday," but once I saw this definition, I thought it was such a perfect word for recovery and sobriety. An intense feeling to make a change is something we all, as addicts, have experienced. I believe we would not be here right now if this were not true. My favorite part of the definition, which surprised me, was the last part: typically something that one has lost. There is no addict in the world who has not regretted losing something from their past once they started using. It is a simple fact of the circumstance.

I wonder when the yearning for change actually begins for an addict? I would have to believe it is personal and individual for everyone depending on their circumstances and reasons for using in the first place. I also have to believe the yearning for change begins long before we recognize it, and therefore, we effectively ignore it for as long as possible. We ignore it because we know with yearning comes work and nothing worthwhile ever comes easy. One of the reasons most of us hide under the clouded veil of our addictions is to avoid the uncomfortable realities of life. Working hard to achieve something not necessarily guaranteed is an uncomfortable notion, and many people shy away, let alone addicts. We couldn't be bothered with dealing with the pains of the actual living world. So we drown them until we can't take it anymore.

When Yearning Becomes a Necessity

At some point, for every single one of us, we hit a point in our downward spiraling journey where we just can't handle the pain we are inflicting on our minds and bodies. When that time finally arrives, the yearning we have been ignoring for years suddenly awakens and becomes so visceral and loud within our minds we can no longer ignore it. In fact, it begins to envelop our every thought and action. We begin to think about nothing other than how to find change. Even when we are using, we are thinking about how to stop. We begin to talk about it with our friends and family. We begin searching online for ways to affect change. We begin to think if we do not change, we will die. To me, this is the point of no return because up until this exact thought, we never really considered the damaging effects of our addiction on our minds and bodies. We just pretended the possibility did not exist. Once it does, the yearning becomes all-consuming.

The yearning to make a change is one of the most powerful feelings I have ever felt. It was the catalyst eventually propelling me out of my past failures and into my present and future successes. It taught me who I am, what I want, and of what I am capable. If it were not for the undying yearn to break free from my self-imposed prison, I would not be here today writing my ninety-ninth blog about how much gratitude I have for my sobriety and my new life.

Pay attention and listen to your inner self. The yearning you feel just may be the most important feeling you have ever felt. It may be trying to tell you something that may forever change your entire life. It may change the way you have viewed your life in the past, how you view your life in the present, and how you will view your life in the future.

Don't forget, this entire blog is founded on the idea of perception. Change how you view yourself, and your view of everything around you will change.

Sober - Day 100

The ABCs of Sobriety

I think I am a pretty intelligent person, most of the time, and I think I at least try to be aware of things happening around me, but today it just occurred to me I am already on the letter Z for the ABCs of Sobriety. What the fuck happened to all those days? I really hope I came up with some good words and ideas for the alphabet relating to recovery and sobriety. I just can't believe I am at day one hundred, which means tomorrow is day 101, and the process of trying to turn all these blogs into a book begins. Wow! This means I essentially wrote a full-length self-help book in three and a half months. Not to mention the novel I am about to complete the first draft of by my birthday next week. Two books in three and a half months. What was my answer for the largest benefit from living a sober life? Time!

Anyway, I suppose I should concentrate on the letter of the day. This one was pretty easy because it is one of the things I noticed pretty quickly after quitting drinking. It was especially true when I began to work toward all the goals I had set for myself in recovery and through my sobriety. In the past, I have always been pretty good at a lot of things. I wrote two books. I wrote, recorded, produced, and played all instruments for a five-song music demo. I raced bicycles and completed century rides and triathlons. I did extensive work in photography. I taught scuba diving for over a decade. Not to mention any number of other ventures I have embarked on throughout my life. I was good at all of them, but here is the thing. I was not great at any of them. Today's word will be the difference between my past attempts and my present and future attempts at success.

Z IS FOR ZEALOUS

Definition: adjective; full of, characterized by, or due to zeal; ardently active, devoted, or diligent (dictionary.com). I can honestly say, in the entirety of my life, I have never approached anything I did with the devoted agency necessary to become great at anything. Until now.

People who know me might argue the above point because they have seen the way I can go after things I like or want. Nevertheless, there is a difference between taking something on as a hobby and actually putting everything you have into something while believing at the deepest recesses of your soul you will become great at it and you will succeed. The latter is from where I am approaching every day, every aspect, and every task I take on in my life. I have wasted too much time and too much of my life doing shit half-assed. It is about time to begin orchestrating the life I want to live and the way

I want to live it. The way I am going to do this is by approaching everything I do with zeal.

How can you tell the difference?

Can you see if someone is acting with a zealous intention or disposition? Can you hear it? I think the only person who can answer this question is the person who is doing it. To me, the experience is like night and day. In my past, I have had moments where I was obsessed with an activity or where I spent an enormous amount of time doing something, but looking back now, it is obvious I was engaging in the activities for external purposes. Whether it was to escape a life I was unhappy with or to gain validation for something I was doing, my motivation was outside myself. I received joy from someone telling me I was good at something or something I did was good. Those comments filled me up and made me feel whole. This is why I was never able to fully realize my potential. I was doing it for the wrong reasons and people.

The difference is from where you receive the joy that fills you up and makes you feel whole. This has taken me forty-eight long years to understand and figure out. Of course, not that I have not figured it all out yet, but it has changed my life in a very short period of time. I now write because I am receiving an extraordinary amount of joy from exploring my mind and the way I think. I enjoy taking the information and transferring it onto a page. I love stringing words together and trying to write sentences and paragraphs that make me feel emotion and pride for how I articulate my thoughts. I have ventured away from photographing people and have found joy in photographing things and trying to find ways to make uncool things look cool in an image. I have proclaimed I will write professionally full-time because I can't think of anything I would rather do to make a living than to work from within my own mind.

The difference is in the reasons why we choose to do the things we do. Now, as adults, we have to make choices to do things for other people all the time, and this is fine. I am talking more about the choices we make about our conscious selves and the choices we make toward our personal growth. Everything we do is a choice on some level. The next time you make a choice to do something for yourself, ask yourself what the motivators were for the choice you made. If other people or things are involved in your answer, I believe it will be more difficult for you to do that thing with zeal. Remove the external things or people from your choice and then look at how it affects your choice. I am willing to bet your choice will change, and you will almost instantly feel better about the choice you make. Most importantly, you may then have a more zealous outlook on how you will approach the endeavor.

Doesn't this make me selfish?

Hell no. I don't know how many times I heard the following saying and thought it was a crock of shit. "You have to love yourself before you can love someone else." I knew I didn't love myself, so I could not allow myself to believe it to be true. But, now that I am walking through this world with open eyes and an open heart, I now see the more I take care of and love myself, the more I am capable of taking care of and loving others. There is no question your ability to love is directly correlated to the amount of love you feel for yourself. The more you love yourself, the more you are able to effectively take on tasks, work, relationships, passions, and life with a zealous vigor you may have never known possible.

With how much zeal have you taken on your decision to quit drinking or other addictions? If you are still struggling, you may be able to find out why when you look at the reasons why you are trying to quit. If it is not for you and you alone, I believe the path will be much more difficult.

Take the time to figure out and find your true reasons why you deserve to quit your addiction, and then you will quit your addiction with zeal.

Sober - Day 101

101 Days of Sobriety

I truly cannot believe I am sitting here typing the words to the blog representing my 101st blog about my sober journey. It feels a little surreal, to be honest, because it was really not that long ago when I was dreading day one. I had absolutely no idea how I was going to pull off a day, let alone a month or three months or 101 days of sobriety. I will say I was dedicated; I really wanted to make a change in my life. I knew it was time to find myself and to give myself the opportunity to start my life with a clean slate and see just how much of what I was capable . As it turns out, I am more capable than I thought. Here is the last blog entry for the compilation of blogs I am going to turn into a book, but my blog journey is far from over. I will continue down this path because I have had a lot of really positive feedback from people who have enjoyed this journey with me. I don't know exactly what the future holds for this blog, but I do know there is one.

I thought for today's post I would spend a little bit of time looking back at this journey and recapping some of the things that have come up along the way. I have a lot of people who are taking the time to go back and start on day one, which has been really inspirational for me. When someone messages me and says they just read a particular day and then tells me something they liked about the blog, it takes me back to what was going on in my mind at that time. It also feels really good to hear people say they relate to things I talked about or how they like the way I approached a certain situation. While I am trying my best to stay away from wanting external validation, knowing people are out there, understanding the reason I started all of this certainly does not impede impending future progress. Every view, comment, and message reinvigorates my resolve to continue my own personal sober journey as well as continue to write about it. Thank you to everyone who has supported this blog.

The Beginning

I remember sitting down to write this blog for the first time. I was in Colorado, and I had quit drinking the day before. I woke up and went down to the lobby with my computer and tried to figure out what I wanted to say. For those of you who don't know, I had fallen away from writing for about six or seven years due to some personal reasons and just never found my way back. The significance of my taking the step to begin writing that day was much larger than any of you were aware because it meant I was stepping back toward fear and confronting it head-on. Making the choice to write on day one aligned with some of the things I have written about throughout this blog. It was a choice I had to ultimately make for me, not for anyone else, and because of this, I have begun a new chapter in my life. In fact, I don't even think it is a new chapter anymore. I think it is a rewrite starting from the day I quit drinking and began writing this blog. The difference in my life today because of quitting and writing is unrecognizable compared to where I may have ended up had I not made the choice to quit and begin writing about this journey.

The Process

Once I started writing, I undoubtedly could not stop. It became something I looked forward to every day, and I still do. I love writing about my thoughts surrounding addiction, and I love learning about myself in the process. Probably the most interesting aspect of this process for me has been how it has lined up with everything my therapist had been trying to teach me for the past year and a half. I understood a lot of what she was trying to convey, I could see it, but I could not put it into practice in my own life until I quit drinking. From the day I quit, everything my therapist had ever told me started to make sense. I walk through life seeing things differently, and therefore I approach them differently as well. As you all know, I have become somewhat obsessed with the idea of perception and how it correlates to pretty much every aspect of our lives. I haven't even touched on the idea of perception to the extent I intend to, but I am looking forward to exploring it further with you.

The Product

By opening up to my inner thoughts and expressing them through writing, I found I have much more to offer than I ever thought. The new perception I have garnered of myself and my abilities has allowed me to push myself every day toward goals I now believe are actually achievable. I decided to write another novel and set a deadline for my birthday three and a half months down the road. My birthday is Thursday, and I will achieve this goal. I applied for and was accepted into an online writing company. I have now written seven online articles. I also took on a ghostwriting job for a man who wants me to help him write his life story memoir. And finally, I will be editing a woman's personal memoir before publication as well. All of these are steps in the direction of my ultimate goal of writing professionally full-time.

I am a living and current example of how one simple idea, action, and choice can change the entire direction of your life. The hardest part was knowing how to recognize that decisive decision when it presented itself. I believe we will all know it when we see it, and I believe we all know which decision to make when it is placed before us. We only have to trust we are courageous, deserving, and ready to take that tiny yet significant step in the positive direction of our life-changing future.

If you do not think you are ready yet, ask yourself this one simple question. "Why am I reading this blog or seeking information regarding sobriety?" The answer: Because you are ready.

Take the step.

PART 4
TERMINATION

PART 1
TERMINATION

EPILOGUE

I truly cannot believe I am sitting here writing the epilogue to my first book on sobriety. I waited to write this portion of the book until I had read and edited all of my blogs and written my reflections for them. I wanted to refresh my memory about my experiences and feelings over the past six and half months before I concluded such a personal and monumental life achievement. You will notice I subtitled the four parts of the book as commitment, process, change, and now termination. These are the four processes of psychotherapy, the last being the most important for sobriety, in my mind. Termination is where I find the deepest level of difference in the way I see how sobriety should end and how others believe it to last forever. For me, I truly believe I am no longer an addict, and I am no longer in recovery. I believe this because I have moved on past the constraints of alcoholism and sobriety. I have reset my past and pushed play on my future. Do not allow yourself to be pinned down to a belief that does not support a thriving future.

It is now time to wrap up my first venture in writing about my successful sober journey. I decided to end with one of my more recent blogs because it sums up my belief about sobriety and the direction I want to focus on moving forward. When I first posted this, it was received with a lot of negative criticism. At first, I was discouraged, but as I continue to unpack and explore the idea of easy sobriety, I am met with less and less confrontation. I think this is because there is some serious validity to it.

Throughout my blogs, you have seen I like to find concepts to write about over a period of time to create a series of writing. In the beginning, I wrote about my beginning journey of sobriety and my day-to-day experiences. Later I spent some time writing about the ABCs of Sobriety, which was fun and forced me to invoke my creative side a little. After that, I wrote about Sobriety Myths and then moved on to the Joys of Sobriety. More recently, I have written about Core Beliefs in sobriety and then Label-Free Sobriety. Lastly, I wrote about Sitting with Discomfort. I enjoy writing blog series because it allows me time to work through different ideas, receive feedback from readers, and most importantly, it reminds me of what I am doing and why I started this journey in the first place.

Last night I asked L about her thoughts on the direction my writing has gone, and we ended up having an insightful conversation about sobriety. Since the beginning of my sobriety blog writing journey, I had been playing with the idea I knew would not be popular with the masses. Because of this, I had not delved into it too much, but I had mentioned it from time to time. After my conversation with L last night, it occurred to me maybe it is time for me to pursue my truest feelings about sobriety, addiction, and mindfulness. Maybe it is time to begin exploring my most honest thoughts about my personal experiences and share them in the hopes others may relate and have the opportunity to experience the same experience I have had in sobriety. Maybe it's time for brutal honesty.

Easy sobriety

In my experience, sobriety has been incredibly easy. I know there are many factors as to why this is the case for me, and this is why I am going to spend some time writing about them. It's important to note though I didn't know my sobriety was easy at first. In the beginning, I just dug into my own personal program and didn't pay much attention to what was happening. As I settled into my sobriety, however, I began craving and seeking more information from others. I wanted to talk with people about sobriety and learn more about how everyone else walked down their own sober paths. What I found was quite shocking to me. I quickly realized most people were not having an easy time with sobriety. The common themes as to why this was the case revolved around struggle, pain, sadness, apathy, and discouragement. Most of the stories I heard were not stories of success and triumph; they were stories of the debauchery that took place before sobriety. The information I was learning about sobriety did not encourage me; it made me sad, it confused me, it made me want to do something to help. I began engaging in activities to help wherever I could. I kept my sober blog going, I started recording podcasts, I hosted online sober meetings, I found other people working in sobriety to do videocast interviews with, I reached out to those seeking help, I did whatever I could to try and be of service to my newfound addiction community.

With all this in mind, a thought began to take shape and has been pestering me for quite some time. I have mentioned it from time to time but have refrained from digging into it deeper because it is a thought my sober community has not received well. While I understand why this is true, I can't help but acknowledge this thought has been hanging around for almost five months now, and it may have some credence in the ever-changing and evolving mystical realm of addiction. The thought that kept forming and badgering me was the thought that sobriety does not have to be difficult. It does not have to be a struggle. It does not have to plague the rest of our lives. The thought that kept forming was, for me, there is such a thing as easy sobriety.

Easy and Hard Sobriety

For anyone who has not experienced easy sobriety, simply hearing those words may conjure up some bad feelings and rightfully so. I do not in any way wish to divide our community by expressing my experiences, opinions, and truths about sobriety. I am aware the potential exists, but I hope everyone is able to keep an open mind toward other's experiences. Support is, after all, the catalyst to successful sobriety.

I support you and your experience; please support me and my experience as well.

Like everything in life, there are always multiple approaches to solving a problem. Mathematics is a great example of how different approaches can have drastically different paths toward the same end result. When given a certain equation to solve, one person may approach the problem from an angle that leads them down a clear and concise path to the final and correct answer. Another person may approach the problem from a different angle, and while they may reach the same correct answer, their path may be much longer, more difficult, and more challenging. I believe the path to sobriety is very similar to a mathematical equation. I will concede immediately, however, not everyone is able to embark on the same path, and the path to sobriety may look a little different for every person. With that said, I believe every path to a solution has multiple alternative paths. Some of those paths may require more time, steps, and patience than others.

I have been fortunate to find a path that has been easy, that has been encouraging, that has been productive, and that has been, dare I say, fun. Please remember we all have our own experiences in life, and while this is only my perspective, I have heard others express similar experiences as well. I hope you will remain open to the idea my experience may not only be possible but plausible for you as well. The path to easy sobriety begins with a choice. It is up to us and us alone how difficult our journey is going to be. As I have said throughout this book, our perceptions of alcohol and the world around us directly shape the experience we have with alcohol and the world. While the idea of easy sobriety may not sit well with you, based on your knowledge and experience, I hope you can at least acknowledge the potential exists. If you do, you have taken the first step toward easy sobriety. If you do not believe easy sobriety is possible, I guarantee with 100 percent certainty it will not be possible for you.

Another way to look at this potentially controversial topic is to ask yourself the following question in regard to easy sobriety. What if it is possible to enjoy easy sobriety? What if your experience and many others' experiences could be easy? What do you have to lose? It could be argued it is damaging for someone to hope for easy sobriety if their experience turns out not to be easy. How is this any different from many of our own personal journeys? We have all encountered letdowns along the way. We have encountered disappointments. We have encountered failures. These are all facts of life and something we either bounce back from or choose to give up on. Taking a chance to change your perception of sobriety does not put you at further risk. At the very least, it offers you a moment to see that there are people out there having different experiences. It allows you to see there are people out there who do not believe you have to be an addict for the rest of your life. It allows you the ability to see something commonly touted as one-dimensional as multidimensional, and you have the power to make the choice. It allows you to choose your own journey.

YOU ARE IN CHARGE OF YOUR JOURNEY

As I wrap up this incredibly powerful venture in my life, I am both humbled and inspired for what is to come. I will undoubtedly continue to write about my sober journey. I will continue writing my novel. I will continue participating in the sober community. I will continue to be here for anyone who needs support while finding their path. I don't really have a choice because it is what I feel compelled to do. What I am more concerned with is what is next for you.

I hope, at the very least, you will let what I have written here simmer. I hope you will look for more books to read about sobriety. I hope you will reach out and find others who are doing what you are doing so you can build a community of support for yourself. I hope you will ask questions and seek answers about the society of alcohol. I hope you will not settle for anything less than what you actually deserve and realize it is much different than what you think you deserve. I hope you will begin new adventures. I hope you will chase your old dreams and create new ones. I hope you will live as we once lived before we were tainted by negativity. I hope you will see there is a strength inside of you waiting for your permission to explode. I hope you will see the strength in others and help them realize their strength as well. I hope you will live as the best version of yourself. I hope for nothing but the absolute best for you.

No matter what happens from this point forward in your journey, I ask one small favor. My therapist said something to me during our journey together, and it hit me very hard. It wasn't what she said about me that hit me hard. What hit me so hard was the idea she could actually believe what she said about me. In response to me stating how I wanted to be a good man, she replied, "You are already a great man." I ask for you to accept the possibility you are already who you want to be; you need only to give yourself permission to begin living as that person.

REFLECTION 1
A SUPPORT NETWORK

The first and arguably most important aspect of easy sobriety came in the form of my support network. This aspect of sobriety can be very different for everyone and especially for those who may feel isolated by their sobriety. It is not uncommon to realize rather quickly your entire network of friends and family are not comfortable with the idea of you trying to live a sober life. Your network can slowly disintegrate and leave you feeling rather isolated. I understand this feeling completely and, if I am truly honest, still deal with it today. Nevertheless, while it may feel like a lonely road, there are options available to us; we just have to be open to them. I found several aspects of support crucial in my sobriety. The first was the support of close family, then opening myself up to new like-minded friends, and finally support in the form of literature and education.

FAMILIAL NETWORKS

I was incredibly fortunate to have had a somewhat built-in support system when my partner and I both decided to quit drinking together. As I wrote in the prologue, we had planned to quit together, but I ended up starting just under two weeks after her. After licking my wounds and pulling up my boots, I finally decided to jump on the bandwagon and join my partner in her successful attempt at sobriety. I will not lie and say I was not terrified to join her but watching her handle her sobriety so well inspired me. She helped to catapult me onto my own path, and then we did sobriety together. This truly was a blessing for both of us. Having not only a friend but a loved one supporting our goals is a gift never to be overlooked, and we haven't overlooked it. To this day, we still talk about how lucky we are to have had each other on this journey.

In the early days of our sobriety, L and I spent a lot of time discussing our experiences of living alcohol-free. I would go so far as to say we actually had fun talking about how different our worlds were becoming and how differently we saw our worlds. Sobriety is not simply not drinking. It is reshaping our minds and bodies to see a life without a chemical whose sole purpose is to suppress our ability to see and feel. The world is crammed with beauty and joys we have hidden from behind the clouded lens of alcohol. L and I were experiencing similar things, and those things incited excitement, and the excitement created questions, and those questions needed to be answered. We bounced ideas off each other. We shared experiences. We asked questions, and then we answered them together. I remember evenings when we got home from work, rather than participating in our regular after-work activities, we ended up sitting down at the kitchen table because one of us had made an observation we couldn't wait to share with the other. Those conversations often turned into an hour or more until one of us realized we had already spent half the evening communicating with each other about how much we were enjoying our newly found sober lives. The conversations with L alone were worth any discomfort we experienced while taking our first steps into sobriety.

Along with our conversations, we found a lot of joy in playing with the idea of mocktails together. If you have not embarked on this activity, I highly recommend it. I will preface this by saying there are a lot of people who believe drinking non-alcoholic drinks is a very bad idea. I respect their opinion but respectfully disagree, as well. For most of us, we indulge in our drinking habits for years upon years upon years. The habitual aspect of addiction is probably the most difficult to curtail for obvious reasons. I think it is unrealistic to expect we could simply walk away from it; the idea is actually quite preposterous. For L and myself, however, we didn't really ever miss the alcohol. What we missed more was the feeling of the glass or can in our hand. We missed the routine of making, pouring, and sharing in the ritual of drinking. We decided, quite quickly, we were not going to let that ritual go, at least for the time being. So, we started experimenting with mocktails, and we had a lot of fun doing it.

In the end, we found some non-alcoholic drinks we liked. L found some dealcoholized wine and champagne that tickled her fancy, and I found some non-alcoholic beer that works for me. We still, to this day, participate in our non-alcoholic happy hours together, and we both very much look forward to the routine of sharing in that ritual together. With over six months sober and an incredibly strong mental attitude against ever drinking again, I feel confident a person can experiment with drinking non-alcoholic drinks without the concern of relapsing. Do not be afraid to be and trust in yourself on this journey because sobriety is probably one of the most personal and individual journeys you can take. What works for one person may not work for another. I have found NA beer to be a lovely replacement, and I have no reservations about continuing to enjoy it as a healthy alternative.

Along with L, we found support in some of our close family too. All of our families knew how much L and I drank, though they never really said anything about it. Nevertheless, they knew. Looking back, I remember feeling self-conscious about how much we would drink while visiting. We would always arrive at a family's house stocked with our wine and beer just in case they did not have any waiting for us. Generally, they would always have something at the ready because they knew we would be looking for it. I figure they bought it for us, so we didn't have to waste time away on our shopping excursions to stock up on alcohol. We usually ended up making runs at some point anyway.

I am sure when they first heard the news of our sobriety, they brushed it off as another J.W. and L escapade, but even then, they were supportive. I was hesitant to even bring it up at first because I knew I had tried and failed in the past. There is nothing worse than someone thinking you are one of those people. You know the people I am talking about, the people who are continually on and off the wagon. I was pleasantly surprised how, when I started bringing up our sobriety, all of our families on both sides were nothing but supportive. I don't recall hearing one disparaging or condescending remark as I had first thought I would. Knowing you have people out there on your side rooting for you is an invaluable asset to sobriety, no matter how you look at it. We were fortunate to have many.

Some of our family have even expressed interest in joining us on our sober journey and that, of course, is wonderful. I have become so involved with the sober community I am happy to talk about and discuss it with anyone at any time. We have had some zoom conversations with family members about sobriety, and we plan on purchasing some new non-alcoholic drinks from a new company in Canada to bring down when we visit them. Hopefully, they will find as much joy in the non-alcoholic idea as we have, and they can use it to help propel themselves onto their own sober journey as well. It is fun and encouraging to share your experiences with people who are close to you.

New like-minded friends

Family is really an integral part of our societal makeup, but not all of us have access to or relationships with our family. Throughout my adult life, the size of my family has dwindled dramatically. The shrinkage of family was not due to loss but more from a loss of touch. As we grow and change, we sometimes grow away from people we were once close to. I don't think I lost touch due to my own personal growth in the beginning, but lately, I certainly think that is more the case. The family I still have are very close to me, and I am very grateful for their place in my life. Interestingly, I have had similar experiences with trying to maintain friends in my life. I have always had a deep-seated desire to have close friends, but I just never seemed to find the right people. Or I was never open enough to have a mutually beneficial relationship. Either way, as I continue to walk down my sober path, I have found a great desire to develop and maintain friendships.

The potential for losing friends along our sober journey is not only possible but very plausible. The shift in mindset following the sober brain is remarkable, and it happens quite quickly. Some of our old friends will understand, relate, and even try to support us on our new journeys. Unfortunately, the majority of our friends, in my experience, do not do this. Alcohol has become so normalized in society people who do not drink are confusing to those who do. There is a quote that fits this situation pretty well: "People are afraid of things they do not understand" (Bill Laswell). When we were immersed in our alcoholic lives, we did not understand sober people either; it's just a fact of the lifestyle. I remember specifically saying things like: "Why would you bother drinking non-alcoholic beer?" As a vegetarian, I have experienced similar reactions to my diet. People just can't understand why a person would choose not to eat meat.

Nevertheless, as our old friends begin to fall away from us, there are, thankfully, numerous avenues available to create new friendships in the world of sobriety. The only caveat to this is you have to be open to recognizing these people when they present themselves to you. You have to be willing to accept your "new" people may not be what you expected. I have experienced this over and over again while on my sober journey. My situation is a little different because I have also fully engaged in the sober community and therefore have more access to a larger group of people than the average person who enters sobriety. Regardless of your access to the sober community, all it really takes is a little awareness. I realized quickly people are around us every day who, by choice, do not drink. I am speaking of those people who have never felt the attraction to alcohol in the first place. It just never had a place in their lives. Can you think of a better type of person with whom to surround yourself in the beginning stages of sobriety?

For me, it turned out my neighborhood held several couples and families who do not drink, and it has nothing to do with having a "problem" with alcohol. They just don't drink. I have learned some of the friends I have known for years don't drink either. I don't know why we don't ever see this while drinking. Open your eyes and pay attention to the people around you. You will be surprised at the community you already have who will support your new way of thinking and your new desire to live alcohol-free.

Aside from the people you already have around you who are sober, once you quit drinking, you are automatically enrolled in a massive community of people who are more supportive and willing to help than you can possibly imagine. The sober community is all around you all the time. The internet offers endless access to alcohol-free support groups, meetings, forums, and resources. In fact, the access is so unlimited it can be overwhelming at first. Take baby steps as you venture into your research about online support communities. I recommend starting with whatever social media platforms you already have. Search hashtags such as #sober, #sobriety, #recovery, #alcoholfree, #teetotaler, #alcohol, #alcoholism, etc. You will have immediate access to more information than you can process. Start with the first thing that catches your attention, and give it a try. Be careful and aware because there are negative resources out there as well. When you find something that works for you, keep it. If you find something that doesn't work for you, toss it.

What I found from my research into the sober community is there are a lot of people who are either passionate about their success or passionate about their process. These people, like me, love to talk about sobriety. They find joy and healing in talking about what is working for them as well as in listening to what works for others. Friendships sprout with little or no effort because there is an immediate connection. The connection is powerful from an emotional and physical level. Nobody understands what you are going through more than someone who is either currently going through it or someone who has successfully experienced it and came out on the other side. Both are beneficial, but I would recommend leaning toward those who have been successful in their sobriety and are willing to help because they feel the drive to do so.

I believe I have already developed some lifelong friendships from my sober journey, and I am grateful for those people. While witnessing people you care about struggle with alcohol can be incredibly frustrating, the successes that eventually follow are powerful on a level I cannot adequately express in words. There is something about being there for someone who just needs a kind word or someone to reach out to. The relationships built through sobriety can and should be mutually beneficial, which is the foundation for the best and strongest relationships we can find. While the beginning steps on your sober journey can feel overwhelming and all-consuming, don't forget to give back to those new relationships and friendships you acquire. We all need kind words, check-ins, and connections no matter where we are on our journey.

LITERARY AND EDUCATIONAL SUPPORT

The last and certainly not least important aspect of support on my journey came in the form of sober literature and knowledge (also known as Quitlit). I have talked a little about this already, but I believe it is important and I want to spend a little more time on this medium of support for the newly sober person. I will speak to my personal experience with Quitlit, but remember, everyone is different, and everyone's journey will be different, so the literature and knowledge that works for you may be different than mine. The important takeaway here is to understand one of the best things you can do in early sobriety is to arm yourself with the knowledge you need to go into battle when the time comes and to emerge victoriously with the help of that knowledge.

As I stated in the prologue, I feel I was very fortunate to have come across the piece of Quitlit I did when I did. Since my partner started her sobriety thirteen days before mine, she had a head start and was already reading literature in an attempt to help facilitate her sobriety. The book she chose to do that with was Annie Grace's *This Naked Mind*. She was wanting to talk with me about what she was reading, but since I was not yet sober, some of what she wanted to discuss with me did not make sense. Looking back now, I am certain it must have been a little frustrating for her. About a week before I quit, I was reacquainted with an old friend whom I referred to as D in the blog. At the time, she was three years sober, and she told me about a book she read at the beginning over a glass of wine that changed her life. The book she was reading while drinking, and this is encouraged in the book, was *This Naked Mind*. I had two recommendations from two people I held a lot of respect for to read the book, so I purchased it with the intent of reading it on day one.

Looking back on it now, it is hard to believe one piece of literature could hold as much power as that book did for me. It was instantaneous. Things just started clicking. All of the thoughts I have had in the back of my head about drinking throughout the years began to make sense. She used science to back up what she preached about alcohol. There were testimonials that read like my autobiography. She broke down the system of alcohol in ways that allowed me to step away from my guilt and fear and allowed me to witness it as a bystander. The book afforded me the confidence to see past my own desires and to see the truth the entire industry of alcohol desperately wants no one to ever see. It allowed me to make my own judgments about why I no longer wanted alcohol in my life, but even more importantly, it gave me a reason to quit alcohol outside the common complaints. Everything I learned from the book was mind-boggling, but the most poignant takeaway from the book for me was the idea I could quit drinking and not miss alcohol in the least. Annie began talking about the ability to do this early in her book, and when you first read it, you are not really sure how to take it. Fortunately, It is true on a level I cannot even adequately express to those who have not experienced it.

Since the 101 Days of Sobriety ended, I have continued writing my blog and podcasting. I have taken the idea of not missing alcohol to new extremes. I have written about my belief there are two types of sobriety: easy and hard. Yes, I just said that one of the types of sobriety is, in fact, easy. This is not met with a lot of warmth in the sober community, and I will not get into the reasons why at this time. Nevertheless, I believe it with such conviction once I am done with this book, I will be venturing into a new project and book to explore the potential for easy sobriety further. Stay tuned.

One of the reasons I believe in the idea of easy sobriety so strongly is because I have witnessed it first hand, and so too has L. We both have similar experiences in this regard, and we both have reasons why we think our journey has been different from others. Both of us attribute some of our ease of sobriety to Annie Grace's book. I will give you a quick run-down of what her book meant to me and my sobriety and encourage you to continue following my journey if you want to learn more about the idea of easy sobriety. The first piece from Annie's book that propelled my desire to quit drinking was when she said, "Alcohol is the only drug you have to make an excuse not to do." I think I repeated it several times before it really clicked, but when it clicked, it pissed me off. I had just experienced a get-together with friends after L and I first quit drinking. We were a little stressed about how to handle the situation with our drinking friends. We were worried about how to act, what to say, what excuse we would use to explain why we, the heavy drinking couple, were not drinking. In the end, I ordered a NA beer and kept the label turned toward me, and L ordered a soda with cranberry. I asked the server to bring it in a cocktail glass. Nobody was the wiser, and we escaped the evening without the barrage of questioning that usually follows someone making a choice not to drink. But that's not the point, is it? Why should we have to stress about hanging out with our friends simply because we have made a choice not to drink? It doesn't make any sense, but it also doesn't make it any less real. The book stating this and experiencing it first-hand made me angry. It lit a fire under me to investigate further the lies alcohol has been telling us.

There are a myriad of options out there for educational support through literature. I found some amazing blogs about sobriety that have been helpful. Following sober support groups on Facebook and Twitter are a resource too. Reading people's posts of struggle and success are constant reminders that can help you remain strong and successful in recovery. As I have said numerous times, what works for you is going to be different and personal to your needs and history. You have to take the time and open yourself up to what may resonate with you so you can grab a hold of them and use them to keep you on your path. Keep your mind open and willing to try new things. Ask for advice from people you trust and or look up to about what has worked for them. Read as much literature as you can about the science behind alcohol and alcoholism. Arm yourself for battle and know the mere act of doing so may ensure you never need to engage in a battle because you are adequately prepared to walk a path of easy sobriety rather than difficult sobriety. It really is up to you, but you have to actively engage in your sobriety and in your journey.

REFLECTION 2
MY THERAPEUTIC JOURNEY

It is an unfortunate and horrifically sad reality to know you drank away thirty years of your life. I am not saying there were no good times during my drinking days, but I am saying what I remember of them is skewed. Not to mention the lack of accomplishments I achieved due to my inability to motivate myself to do anything other than get through a day of work and to my first drink. The first time you actually realize how much time you have wasted, you involuntary want to reach for a drink. It is about as traumatic a realization as you can make. When you get past the initial shame of it, it begins to get easier, but you will never really get past it fully because it is just too much of a kick in the face. I feel it from time to time when I am reflecting on how far I have come and how much better I am living my life. I think to myself, "Damn, can you imagine where I would be if I would have found sobriety earlier?" It's mind-boggling, but it doesn't change the fact those years are gone, and the only thing left to do is live well moving forward in the hopes of making up for lost time.

As I said earlier, making the connection I needed to quit drinking did not equate to my quitting alcohol. It took many, many more years to figure my shit out. It started with the idea of moderation. I know I can quit if I want to. Have you ever said that to yourself? With that mentality, I tried everything I could think of to moderate my drinking. Drinking every other day. Only drinking on the weekends. Allowing myself only two drinks and then stopping. The attempts go on and on, and all end with the same result: my continued drinking. Nothing worked because, as an addict, I became very good at justifying why it was okay to drink. It's uncanny, really, just how good we can get at justifying our drinking. Once I finally admitted to myself moderation wasn't working, I again made the decision to give therapy a try. I had sought out and tried therapy on several occasions in my past as a way to deal with my issues. It never really worked, and I knew exactly why. I don't do well with placation or passive-aggressive modalities. If, as a therapist you let me, I would figure out how to only tell you what was necessary to keep the conversation going without you ever really catching on to the real me. I was good at it. I needed someone who could see through my bullshit and call me on it. As you have undoubtedly discerned from my blogs, I had multiple addictions. Alcohol, nicotine, and other behaviorally related issues keeping me from living the life I wanted to live, and I was tired of it.

After looking inexhaustibly, I finally found someone who seemed to fit what I was looking for, so I called and made an appointment. The therapist called me back and told me her client list was full and asked if she could refer me to another therapist she knew. I reluctantly agreed. Shortly after, a woman called and introduced herself to me as the therapist referred to by my original pick. We had a short conversation, and I had a decent feeling about her, so I scheduled an appointment. There has never been a more salient decision in my life than the decision to begin seeing the woman who became my therapist.

After the first session, I knew this was the person who was going to allow me to open up in the way I needed to in order to uncover the truths that kept me stuck in my stagnant life. I don't know how I knew it, but I knew it like I have never known anything before. What I didn't know was that the next year and a half was going to be an arduous and even tumultuous time in my road to recovery. What I didn't know was it was going to be a time of deep reflection, understanding, and an uncomfortable uncovering of my truest self. What I didn't know was I was about to embark on a life-altering journey that would forever change my life. I remember having a feeling at one point in my therapeutic journey I was in for a bumpy ride. What I remember even more was for the first time in my life, I didn't care. I was ready and willing to take the ride. It helped, of course, to have the right guide to help me along the way.

When I told my therapists about my addictions and the concerns I had with how much time they were taking up in my life and how much depression they were causing me, she asked one simple question. I didn't understand the significance of this question until later, but when I finally did, everything became even clearer. She asked, "What do you see yourself doing with your time if you are not doing the things you want to stop doing?" It's a simple question, right? While I didn't understand the significance at the time, my answer was immediate and without hesitation. I said, "I would read more, write, do more photography, and exercise more." I think my therapist even chuckled a little at the speediness and specifics of my response. She told me it seemed pretty clear what I wanted; all we needed to do was find a way to get me there. That was the beginning of my therapeutic journey.

I won't take up a lot of time talking about the specifics of my therapy, but I do want to touch on some aspects of my therapy that are still important to me to this day. I never really understood the idea of a "toolbox" for dealing with life. I had heard it a hundred times, but it always sounded pretty idiotic to me. In my mind, before therapy, you didn't need tools to deal with life; you just lived and dealt with the repercussions later; you can see how well this worked for me. The toolbox I intentionally put together while in therapy has opened up doors I never knew existed. The tools I use on a daily basis keep me focused, productive, true to myself, and accountable. I look at my toolbox as my survival kit. I rely on it now like I rely on air. I have too much history living life on a whim to take for granted the positive direction my life has taken. I carry my toolbox with me every day, and I use it unsparingly.

Positive self-talk

The first tool in my toolbox is the notion of using positive self-talk as often and consistently as possible. It is interesting I chose to start with this one because it was honestly the hardest one for me to come by. My therapist and I had a running inside joke during sessions. I would make a comment, and she would give me this scowling look that told me I was doing it again, the negative self-talk. I was a master at it. I could find any reason and any topic to talk down to myself or simply take credit away from something I had done. It was as normal and involuntary as breathing. The negative self-talk went on through the better part of a year until I finally made the decision to quit drinking. With that decision, for reasons I can only surmise, I began to see myself differently, and I began to talk about myself differently, too. It was a welcomed and refreshing change.

The difference between talking negatively about yourself and talking positively about yourself is simply perspective. How you see yourself is how you project yourself onto others. When I was drinking, using nicotine, and engaging in addictive behaviors, I saw myself as a failure and someone who did not deserve happiness. What did I put out into the universe? Exactly those things. What did I receive back from the universe? Exactly those things. I expected bad things to happen, so bad things happened. I expected things not to go my way, so things did not go my way. I expected myself to barely get by, so I barely got by. Immediately upon quitting drinking, nicotine, and negative behaviors, I began to feel deserving of more. I began to feel I could do more. I began to feel there was more available to me than what I had allowed myself to see. I began to feel worthy of a good life. What has happened as a result? I began to receive good things. I am doing the things I have wanted to do for years. I am living well and achieving my goals. I am living my best life. What is the biggest difference? My perspective changed. I no longer saw myself as the person I was while drinking. I saw myself as somebody completely different and completely worthy, and therefore, I was and am worthy.

It is a difficult change to make for someone who grew up talking negatively about themselves for decades. It requires some practice, discipline, and accountability. It is so much easier to fall back into the old comfortable way of life when times get tough. But you have to push through. It does get easier. In the beginning, I found myself making statements to myself I didn't even believe, but they were statements I wanted to believe. I knew I had to keep repeating them over and over until I started to believe them. It took a while, and at first, I didn't know if it would ever actually work. It did. I started to believe the positive statements I told myself. One by one, I began to see and believe those statements until eventually, every positive statement I made about myself sounded real, sounded true, sounded like me. I effectively talked myself into a new perspective. You can, too.

Sitting with Discomfort

One of the biggest obstacles I see and hear people struggle with in sobriety is how to deal with discomfort. The discomfort can be bad news, cravings, or just a bad day. When we, as addicts, do not feel good, we use our addiction to numb or neutralize that feeling. We don't know how to do anything else. There are a couple of steps I now use as a way to deal with bad feelings or discomfort. The first is to recognize the craving, need, or desire.

If we do not recognize and accept what is happening, we cannot effectively deal with it. We will turn to our reactionary survival skills and do what provides the most instant gratification. Our addiction. It's almost involuntary at this point; we have programmed our bodies to believe it needs the substance we have become addicted to. But guess what? There is a reason we have evolved the way we have. We have the mental capacity to think past our immediate and instinctual desires and needs. We do not need to act on instinct alone.

What does it mean to recognize the craving or need? It's simple. You know that feeling you have when something really good or pleasurable happens for you? Picture the warmth you feel in your chest, the smile that spreads across your face, the lightness you feel in your body, and the overwhelming sense you can do no wrong? Remember that feeling? It's visceral, consuming, and overwhelming, isn't it? Now, picture the feeling that accompanies craving. Visualize your heartbeat as it escalates. Feel the clamminess of your skin. Remember the difficulty you have taking in a full breath. See the scattered thoughts swimming through your mind. Feel the panic swelling inside your chest. Recognize the irritability taking over your entire body. Can you picture it? Good, then you can recognize it when it occurs again.

Why is it important to recognize this feeling when it occurs? Recognition is the opposite of reaction. When we react to a situation, we are skipping the step of recognition. This step buys us a little time to consider our options. When we skip this step, we severely limit our options for action. Try and remember a time when you lashed out at someone or something. Can you remember that feeling of instant reaction? Do you also remember the guilt that followed? Generally, when we react without consideration, we regret the outcome. This is because we did not consider all the consequences of our actions. We simply went with our instincts, and in a civilized setting, our instincts do not benefit us the way they did our cave-dwelling ancestors. The same is true with the discomfort of cravings. If we do not recognize them and consider the repercussions of our actions, we will most likely regret our decisions.

The next step is acknowledging the discomfort. This sounds similar to the first step, but it is quite different. Recognizing the craving and discomfort is just taking a moment to realize there is a reason why we are not feeling good or normal. We recognize something is going on in our minds and bodies and we do not like the feeling. Rather than simply doing what we usually do, try to numb the feeling, we instead take a moment to understand from where the feeling is coming and the need to address it. Acknowledging the discomfort is the most deliberate part of this technique. Acknowledging the discomfort means we are actively engaging with them by saying to ourselves, or out loud if we wish, we see the craving. That sounds a little weird but bear with me.

I remember when I first went to therapy and outlined some of the addictions and issues I wanted to deal with, one of them was personal, and I asked my therapist if it was going to be okay with her. Her response was she looked at people's issues, addictions, emotions, etc., like separate and individual "things" that require attention on a therapeutic level but the actual 'things' themselves were not where the focus was placed. The focus was placed on the understanding of those "things" from an emotional standpoint, how to change the way we perceived them, and how they affected our lives. This stuck with me throughout the entirety of my therapeutic journey.

The next step is to visualize the discomfort. When acknowledging the discomfort associated with the cravings or bad feelings, I began to view them as separate 'things' I could visually see, and I let them sit there (quite literally) out in front of me. By watching my feelings out in front of me, I am able to acknowledge them but not give them any real credit. I take power away from them because they are not part of me; they are separate from me. I don't know how to adequately describe the way I visualize those feelings, but they are colors and shapes. They start out red, orange, and yellow, and they swirl around quickly in the beginning. The longer I sit there observing the feelings, the cooler their colors become. They begin to move slower and slower until, eventually, they disappear completely. Once the feelings of craving and discomfort have dissipated, I re-engage with my day feeling more confident, happy, and accomplished. I feel proud of myself because I did not give in to the feelings of discomfort repeatedly trying to throw me off my path.

Living with intention

I don't know what possessed me to take on the tasks I took on when I began my sober journey, but I am glad I did for many reasons. I knew part of what drove my desire to drink and use was boredom. I had settled, begun to live a stagnant life, and had little energy to take on new adventures. I did, however, have plenty of desire to indulge in libations. I knew I needed to seek out ways to entertain myself and my time. What I didn't know was by doing so, I was setting myself up for a life full of intention. This intention would engulf every aspect of my being and virtually ensure not only the success of my sobriety but the success of my life as well. Since beginning my sober journey, I have embarked on a life of intention I look forward to every day. I seek out and find challenges. I am living the life I always thought I deserved but never knew I could have. Here is how I began living with intention.

The first thing I did was choose to begin educating myself. By doing so, I unintentionally began donning the armor I unknowingly needed to easily combat the struggles associated with the cessation of addiction. I made a point to read every day about the chemicals plaguing me for the better part of my entire life. I learned why they did what they did to my mind and body. I learned how they negatively affected me and everyone around me. I learned how I unintentionally developed a dependency on those chemicals but also how I could remove the dependency. I learned the reason I felt miserable in my "comfortable life" was due to the breakdown of my emotional and physical self at the hands of different forms of poison. I learned I had the power to change, and I took the power and began making changes.

The second thing I did was choose to be present in my life. For anyone suffering from addiction, you know what it means to be absent from life. We choose our addictions over things that really matter: our jobs, families, friends, hobbies, and passions. We disconnect from what essentially makes life worth living. Since I became sober, I have been more present for my family and friends. I laugh more, probably because I pay better attention. I play with my son more. I communicate with L better. I am better at my job. I am enjoying my time with even mundane things more. I am better at living life because I am present and aware. This affords me the ability to offer more than I take from this life. That, unbeknownst to me, is one of the best parts of living, but I was just too busy disconnecting to see it.

The third thing I did was engage in one of my past loves, writing. I vowed to write every day about my experiences with sobriety. At first, I vowed to write every day for thirty days. Then, when the first thirty days were over, I vowed to write for 101 days. When those days were over, I vowed to keep writing, and here I am. I am writing about my sober journey, and it has been the single greatest gift I have ever given myself. Since vowing to write about my journey, I have decided to turn my first 101 days of sobriety into this book, I have written a full-length novel, I have begun a sobriety podcast, I am doing videocasts with other like-minded people, and I have made the decision to take my greatest passion and turn it into my career. Every day, I wake up clear-headed and ready to engage in my life of intentions.

Since I wrote my 101 days of sobriety and began turning them into this book, I have learned about and found a myriad of new tools to place in my emotional toolbox. In an effort to remain true to the first 101 days of my sobriety, I would have to say these three tools were the first and most influential in my sober journey.

The last twenty-six days of my 101-day journey went in an entirely different direction. Looking back, I believe I wanted to engage my more creative side during this time period. I decided to write the last twenty-six days as an ABCs of Sobriety series. The idea was to pick a word for each letter of the alphabet and then write about my experience with the word while on my sober journey. This series was a lot of fun for me to write, and I still remember the day I wrote Z and recognized how fast the last twenty-six days flew by. It was incredible, and it showed me just how powerful writing was for my recovery. I look back at the last twenty-six days of my 101 days of sobriety with complete and utter fondness. I hope you will, too.

RESOURCES

Where to find me:

Website:	https://xstopwriting.com
Sober Militia Blog:	https://xstopwriting.com/sobermilitia
Sober Militia Podcast:	https://xstopwriting.com/podcast

- Also available on Spotify, Apple Podcasts, Google Podcasts, Anchor FM

VideoCast Interviews: https://xstopwriting.com/videocast

Social Media

Instagram:	https://instagram.com/xstopwriting
Facebook:	https://facebook.com/xstopwriting
Twitter:	https://twitter.com/xstopwriting

Sober Facebook Group

Sober Militia:
https://facebook.com/groups/sobermilitia2020

Recommended Reading

This Naked Mind by Annie Grace
We Are the Luckiest by Laura McKowen
Quit Like a Woman by Holly Whitaker

Alcohol Explained by William Porter

The Secret Life of a Hollywood Sex and Love Addict by Brianne Davis

Mommy Drunkest by Brittany Priestley

Indulge in Mocktails by Carmell Pelly

J.W.'S CORE SOBRIETY TIPS

After writing the first 101 Days of Sobriety, I continued writing my blogs and added podcasts as well. Throughout my continued journey to find the possible reasons for easy sobriety, I have uncovered many beliefs and aspects of living I feel are paramount for successful sobriety. From the more than two hundred blogs I have written since the first 101 days, I chose three of them to share with you because I believe them to be the most inspirational and helpful for me. I hope they are for you as well. If you like the first paragraph included here, please follow the included link to read the blog in its entirety.

FINDING OUR WHYS

As many of you know, I spend a lot of time reflecting on my sober journey. More specifically, I spend a lot of time trying to understand the differences between my journey and other people's journeys. From day one of sobriety, it became clear to me that not all paths are created equal. For some, the journey is incredibly difficult and lifelong. For others, the journey is a struggle but a struggle with an end in sight. Still, others experience the journey as simply a hopeful survival from one day to the next. Occasionally, you will hear about a journey with far fewer obstacles, struggles, and dependencies on things outside our control. It is these rarer occasions I find the most intriguing. I am intrigued by these journeys partly because it is how I found my experience to be, but it is also because I am obsessed with why there is such a disparity in the difficulty of experiences from one person to the next. How can one person experience such pain and torment on their path while another can experience ease and grace? I believe the answers lie in the whys.

To read this blog in its entirety, follow this link to my website and blog: https://www.xstopwriting.com/post/finding-our-whys

Label-Free Sobriety

A close friend of mine, Bobby C., brought up this idea to me the other day and I have been stewing on it for the better part of a couple weeks. He asked the following question: "What would happen if we didn't label ourselves in sobriety?" It didn't hit me right away, but later it occurred to time that labels make up a large portion of why we do almost everything we do. Think about it. Husband/wife, straight/gay, male/female, skinny/fat, young/old, blue-collar/white-collar, rich/poor, BMW/Hyundai, drunk/sober, and the list goes on and on and on and on. Everything we do has a label attached to it where there does not always need to be one. Does it really matter if I am the husband or the wife in a relationship? Does it really matter if I am male or female? Does it really matter what kind of car I drive? The only time it really matters is when you are asked to state the information on a form or as an answer to a question. In the end, the only weight the information carries is the weight we, the person stating the information, give it. Otherwise, it is just a man-made label.

To read this blog in its entirety, follow this link to my website and blog: https://www.xstopwriting.com/post/label-free-sobriety

Perpetuate Positive Sobriety

As many of you know, my experience in sobriety has been incredibly positive. It has been so positive, I have dedicated a large portion of my life to helping others experience something similar. The one criticism I have about the sober community is the overabundance of negativity regarding recovery. I have stated this many times in the past, but I do not believe it can be stated too much or too often. We project the outcome of our sobriety. Whether it is a positive or negative projection begins in our thoughts, beliefs, and words. If we say it sucks, it sucks. If we say it's easy, it's easy. We can experience one or the other or any myriad of experiences in between. It's a choice; we choose our experiences every single moment of every single day. We choose via our thoughts, actions, words, beliefs, and even friendships and relationships. Every single one of the before-mentioned provisions comes with options and, therefore, choices. How we choose those options determines the outcome of our moments, days, weeks, years, and lifetimes. It can be difficult to hear how much of a role we play in the outcome of our lives but make no mistake; we play a starring role.

To read this blog in its entirety, follow this link to my website and blog: https://www.xstopwriting.com/post/perpetuate-positive-sobriety

ABOUT THE AUTHOR

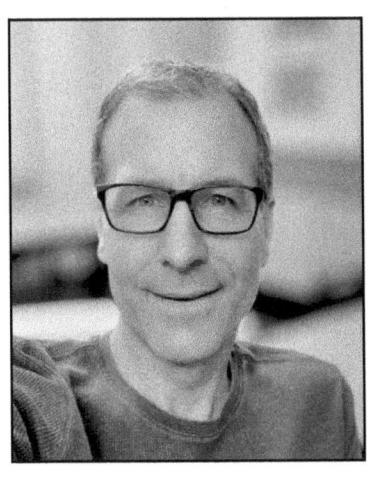

J.W. Collier is a father, partner, author, blogger, podcaster, teacher, and football coach living in the beautiful Pacific Northwest. He found his calling for writing after taking the giant life-step of quitting nicotine and alcohol. He quickly found, after quitting drinking, a large disparity between his experience and the experience of other people in sobriety. Most people tout sobriety as excruciatingly difficult. He found sobriety to be quite easy. Because of this, he made it a life goal to try and find ways to articulate the difference between easy and hard sobriety. One of the ways he is attempting to do this is with his first book, *Alcohol-Free, Straight Up with a Twist*. In this book, J.W. chronicles his journey of sobriety from day one after quitting drinking. He decided to write a blog to help keep him accountable and nothing has been the same ever since. He found not only a passion for people in sobriety but also a passion for writing. Since blog one, he has continued to write his blog, The Sober Militia Blog, record podcasts, conduct videocast interviews with other people in sobriety, write books on sobriety, and run an online sober group.

Next, he will take his experience to the next level and write a follow-up book titled, *Easy Sobriety* in which he will outline the reasons why he believes sobriety has been perpetuated as hard for far too long. J.W. believes there are other ways to approach sobriety that do not require life-long labels, such as "addict" and "in recovery." He believes a person can graduate out of recovery and into a life of normalcy. J.W.'s views on sobriety are not of the norm. He believes choice and perception are the keys to unlocking the potential for easy sobriety. J.W. thinks a person need only believe easy sobriety to be plausible for it to be possible.

REVIEWS

"The way J.W. details his real-time thoughts and inner dialogue during his first 101 days without alcohol is so powerful. Everyone who begins a journey to stop drinking needs to feel less alone, and J.W.'s honest and vulnerable sharing and beautiful insights shine a brilliant light that illuminates the path for others."
 —Annie Grace
 Author of *This Naked Mind* and *The Alcohol Experiment*
 press@thisnakedmind.com
 https://instagram.com/thisnakedmind

"This is a powerful book that takes readers on a journey from the initial uncertainty and fear of day 1, right through to the joys of living a life without alcohol. Raw, real, honest, and emotional at times, *Alcohol-Free* is a must-read for anyone navigating the world of alcohol-free living."
 —Simon Chapple
 Author of *The Sober Survival Guide* and *How to Quit Alcohol in 50 Days*
 Website - www.besober.co.uk
 Instagram: https://instagram.com/besoberandquit
 info@besober.co.uk

"Even though I'm not an alcoholic, I can relate to J.W. Collier's *Alcohol-Free: Straight Up with a Twist*'s story of addiction in this unique glimpse inside the mind of a functioning alcoholic willing to change his life. I applaud anyone willing to admit to their -ism and transform their life."
 —Brianne Davis
 Actress, History Channel's *Six*, and author of best-selling novel *Secret Life of a Hollywood Sex & Love Addict*
 https://instagram.com/thebriannedavis
 secretlifepodcast@icloud.com

"As addicts and alcoholics, our own life experiences lead us down different paths to self-destruction. As we seek our own recovery, we also rediscover who we really are, deep under the alcohol and drugs we drowned ourselves in. No paths are exactly the same, but we all come crashing to a dead end. *Alcohol-Free* is a book of the road not often traveled toward recovery. On Collier's daily trek through sobriety and self-discovery, it feels as if we are growing right along with him. The pages are filled with wisdom and valuable, life-saving insight. I honestly feel his journey can help others who may not be inclined to take alternative routes to recovery. No matter which way we decide to go, towards the betterment of ourselves and those around us, all paths lead to freedom. I know *Alcohol-Free* will help many to find it."
—Brittany Priestley
Author of *Mommy Drunkest*
brittpriestley27@gmail.com
https://instagram.com/brittpriestley27

"The opposite of addiction is not sobriety; the opposite of addiction is connection." —Johan Hari.
"*Alcohol-Free: Straight Up With a Twist* is a detailed, touching, and extremely relatable description of one man's personal journey of sobriety. Whether you have 30 years, 2 years, 30 days, or are simply sober-curious, you will get something out of this book. The author is brutally honest in his writing and does not shy away from detailing every part of his experience in his first 101 days of sobriety.
"*Alcohol-Free* provides a unique insight not only into why someone might decide to become sober but also how to manage the inevitable emotional rollercoaster that will follow, providing teachable moments for maintaining sobriety, perception and living in gratitude. I definitely learned a few things from reading this book!"
—Leah Martin-Brown
Singer-Songwriter at Evol Walks
leahmartinbrown@gmail.com
Instagram: https://instagram.com/adventuresinplasticland

"In J.W. Collier's *Alcohol-Free: Straight Up with a Twist*, we get an honest, raw and vulnerable look at his young beginnings with alcohol. We all have different reasons for drinking, whether early or later in life. J.W. has a way of relating that makes his story something we can all learn from. It's really a story of how you can change, let go of the illusion of alcohol and find real peace and authentic freedom. This book is a great read for anyone on the path to find identification, practical insight, and or who is just "sober curious". Thanks, J.W. for sharing your story and gift of writing with the world."
—Jenn Kautsch (aka SoberSis)
enn@sobersis.com
https://instagram.com/sobersis

"*Alcohol-Free: Straight Up With a Twist* takes us on an exploratory journey of the first 101 days of sobriety with honesty, empathy, and education. You will gain a greater insight into this world and along the way learn about the ABCs of sobriety. A must-read for anyone looking for support or who is sober curious and thinking about taking that next step."
—JoAnne Reynolds
CEO Sexy AF Spirits
Jo@sexyafspirits.com
https://instagram.com/sexyafspiritsjo

Alcohol Free: Straight Up With a Twist is an intimate look into one man's journey to sobriety. I related to J.W.'s persistence and positive perspective. I truly enjoyed his process and his celebration of an alcohol-free life! If you want to feel inspired and motivated to appreciate all the wonders that sobriety brings to life, read this book!"
—Tracie Hutchins
Model and Creator at Sexy is Sober
hutchinsdesign@gmail.com
https://instagram.com/sexy_is_sober

Lightning Source UK Ltd.
Milton Keynes UK
UKHW020155280122
397834UK00003B/132